THE WORLD OF
HAIR

A Scientific Companion

'Who would use this book?'

'Why of course ... you would!'

'So what's so special about this?'

'Ah! This is a journey into hair with its little twists and trails leading you into fascinating things on how to keep hair looking its best.'

'What can it tell me?'

'Many things ... you may have forgotten them or put to one side ... but after reading this you can always let your clients know just how knowledgeable you really are.'

'Will this make me a better hairdresser?'

'That's up to you ... but it will probably make your clients feel better that they're in good hands!'

Alan Goldsbro
Chief Executive, Hairdressing Training Board

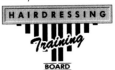

THE WORLD OF
HAIR

A Scientific Companion

DR JOHN GRAY

Contributors

R. Dawber

Consultant Dermatologist, Oxford, UK

C. Gummer

Senior Research Fellow, Procter & Gamble UK

Sponsors

Procter & Gamble Haircare Research Centre

Rusham Park, Egham, Surrey, UK

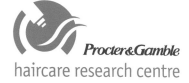

in association with the

Hairdressing Training Board

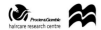

First published 1997 by
MACMILLAN PRESS LTD
Houndmills, Basingstoke, Hampshire RG21 6XS
and London
Companies and representatives
throughout the world

ISBN 0–333–71958–1

A catalogue record for this book is available
from the British Library.

This book is printed on paper suitable for recycling and
made from fully managed and sustained forest sources.

10   9   8   7   6   5   4   3   2   1
06 06 04 03 02 01 00 99 98 97

Printed in Great Britain by
Jarrold Book Printing, Thetford, Norfolk

Hairdressing Training Board/Macmillan
Series Standing Order ISBN 0–333–69338–8

You can receive future titles in this series as they are published
by placing a standing order. Please contact your bookseller or,
in case of difficulty, write to us at the address below with your
name and address, the title of the series and the ISBN quoted
above.

Customer Services Department, Macmillan Distribution Ltd,
Houndmills, Basingstoke, Hampshire RG21 6XS, England

The author

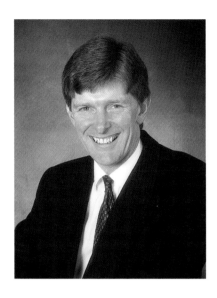

Dr John Gray is a partner in a large group practice and has a long-standing interest in skin and hair problems. He is a Consultant to Procter & Gamble and is involved in their hair education programme. He has lectured widely on the subject of hair health to doctors and hairdressers.

He has recently been elected to the membership of the European and American Hair Research Societies and of the Royal Society of Medicine.

The contributors

Dr Christopher Gummer gained his doctorate studying genetic and acquired hair diseases. He is currently the Senior Research Fellow at Procter & Gamble, leading hair and skin research in the U.K. and Europe.

Dr Rodney Dawber is Consultant Dermatologist and Clinical Senior Lecturer in Dermatology at the University of Oxford. He is the editor and writer of many textbooks in the fields of hair and nail disorders. He is a founding member of the European Hair Research Society and is recognised as one of the leading hair experts in the world.

Acknowledgements

My thanks to:

Dorte and Kristiana for their support, help and advice,
Janet Smith for her indefatigable efforts in typing and organisation,
Jean Macqueen (my editor), Vidal Sassoon Salons, London, and
Collections Hair Club, Weybridge, Rodney Dawber and
Christopher Gummer for their expertise, support and encouragement,
Rodney Dawber and David Whiting for provision of materials,

and

all those kind people whom I accosted in the street and who allowed me
to photograph their hair in order to make this book happen.

This book attempts to look at the normal hair around us –
both good and bad.

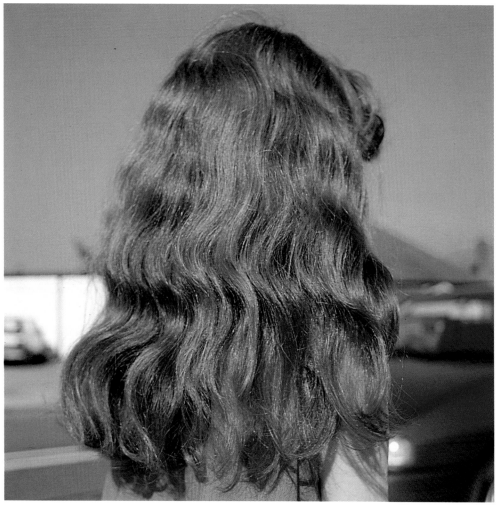

'Fair tresses man's imperial race ensnare
and beauty draws us with a single hair.'

Alexander Pope, 1688–1744

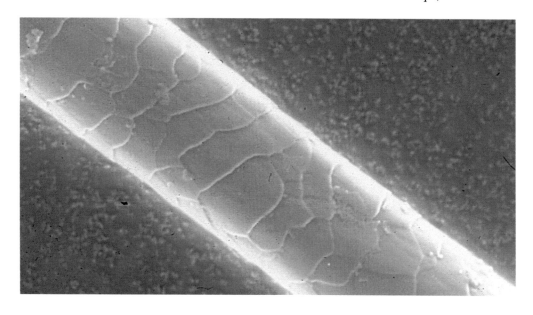

Contents

Introduction

Why *another* book about hair?

People all over the world see hair as important. In the west, for instance, almost all brides are prepared for their approach to the altar by the hands of an expert stylist. On that supreme day, their hair style may be the most elaborate they will ever have in their lives. At the opposite extreme, when a young girl of one of the aboriginal tribes of the Amazon jungle reaches puberty the women of the village ceremonially remove all the hairs from her head, one by one. The ritual significance and mystique of hair on these occasions are undeniable.

We use our hair to express our personalities – to conform, to make a statement, to help us feel good, to attract other people. Sometimes our hair even seems to reflect our mood, especially when we are sad or depressed.

Our hair is perhaps our most distinctive feature. Any sudden change in its colour or style startles our friends and produces comments from our family.

Hair is an amazing material. In the hands of an expert and with the use of modern hair care products, it is soft and shining and seems full of life. Strangely, however, hair is *dead*.

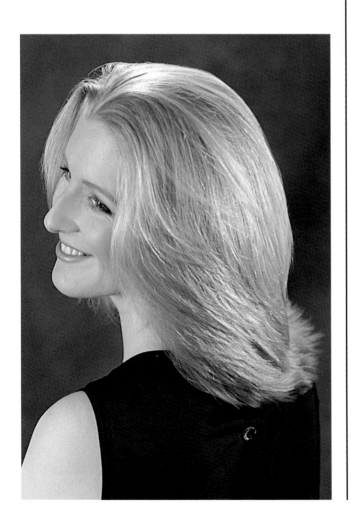

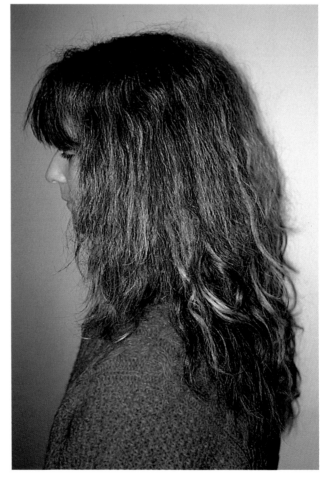

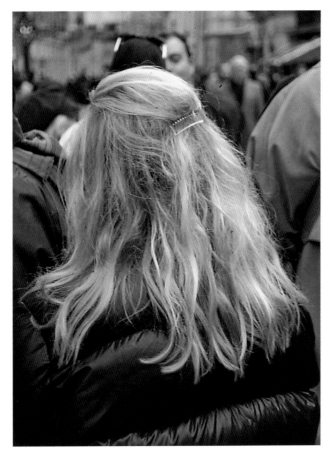

Neglected hair!

Hair, like beautiful wood, can be shaped, moulded, coloured and, if properly looked after, made to shine with 'health'. Yet all too often this 'crowning glory' of ours is neglected. And then it can look shoddy, dull and lifeless. It becomes a constant disappointment, all the worse because we know that, however expensive and beautiful our clothes, if our hair looks a mess we won't be seen as well-groomed, poised and fashionable.

Hair so often fails to do for us exactly what we expected. Its behaviour raises endless questions, sometimes almost despairing:

- *Why* did my hair suddenly collapse just before that vital interview? What could I have done to avoid that happening?
- *Why* did it look fine when I walked out of the salon yesterday, and terrible this morning?
- *Why*, when it had so much volume and 'body' when I was on that Mediterranean holiday, has all that gone now I'm at home in November?

- *Why* were the results of that home colour so disappointing?
- *Why* does a woman's hair so often 'fall out' after she has had a baby?
- *Why* do so many men (and some women) go bald?
- *Why* does so-and-so's lovely red hair never perm very well?
- *Why* does my hair go out of condition so easily? What can I do to restore it?

This book sets out to answer questions like these – the questions hair stylists are asked every working day. Understanding hair from the scientific standpoint helps them to predict what will happen to different types of hair under different conditions. It also allows them to understand what can be done with a particular person's hair and what cannot: every experienced stylist and technician knows how important it is *not* to try to do the impossible with hair that is too thin, too short, the wrong colour or just 'difficult'.

In this book we explore the nature of hair, its care and maintenance, and the cosmetic and medical problems which can and (often do) affect it. Above all, we point to the ways in which the individual, the hair care industry and the hair stylist can work together to create 'healthy hair'.

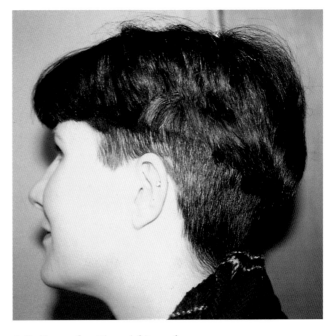

A tinting and cutting nightmare!

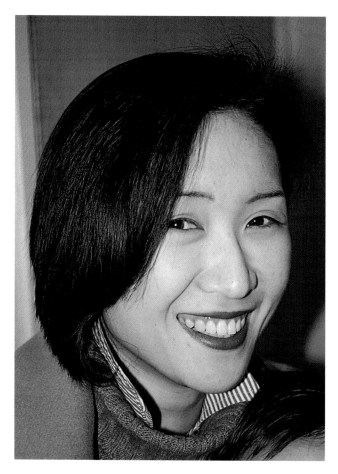

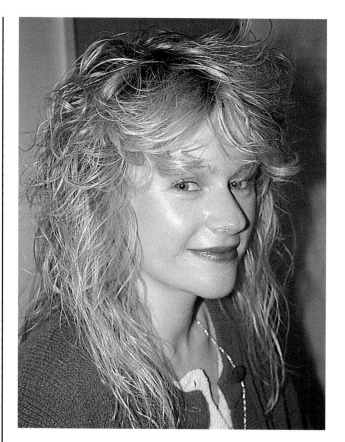

Women from all around the world choose hair styles to suit their type of hair. Hair reflects our personalities, whichever race we come from

The book has been written with the collaboration of scientists working in hair research, doctors, stylists and hair technicians. It is not meant to replace the many existing excellent textbooks on cutting, styling, client care and business management, fields which are rightly those of hairdressing boards, colleges and schools, and salon owners.

It aims to be the most comprehensive illustrated publication available on the basic science of hair and the application of that science in the home and the salon. The writer hopes that it will inform and help all those who work with hair.

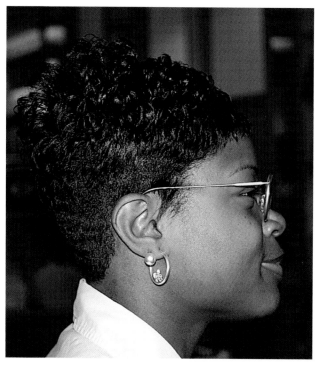

Hair

About this chapter ...

In this chapter we look at the basic properties of hair, how it grows, and why it differs so much from one person to another.

We explain why the quality and quantity of hair changes with the passing of time, and what decides how well it can be styled or cosmetically changed.

Human hair

The hair we have

All land mammals – including humans – have hairy skins, although in us most of the hair is not immediately visible. As with other mammals, our hair characteristics are inherited directly from our parents. Your hair colour and hair type were decided for you, as were the colours of your eyes and your skin.

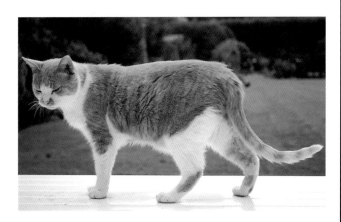

Cats' hair insulates their bodies and may also help them to identify each other

In the end, whether or not your hair has the precious quality of being 'easy to manage' depends on what your parents have passed on to you from your ancestors.

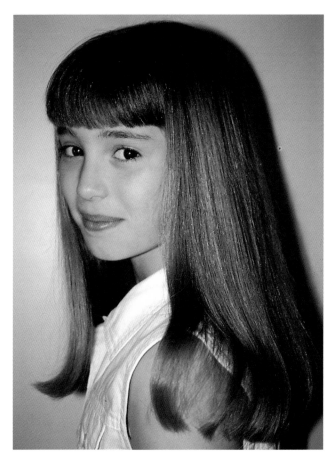

The human 'kitten' has more hair per square centimetre of her skin than the real one, only most of it is too fine to see

What hair does

Scientists believe that hair has evolved for the identification of individuals, and for sexual or status display to other members of their species.

HAIR FACTS

Hair distribution

Humans are covered all over in hair, except on the palms of the hands, the soles of the feet, and the lips.

Hair is most obvious on the head and face (including the nose and ears in some people), the armpits, the groin, and (in men) the chest and legs.

How much hair do we have?

- On average, each person's head carries about 100,000 hair follicles. Some people have as many as 150,000.

- On a baby's head, there are about 1,100 follicles per square centimetre.

- By the age of 25, this number has fallen to about 600, but the number depends on the physical type of the individual.

- Between the ages of 30 and 50, the number drops further, to 250–300. There is only a slight further fall with age.

- Each follicle grows about 20 new hairs in a lifetime. Each new hair grows for several years, and can reach over a metre in length.

- Each hair falls out eventually, and is replaced by a new one.

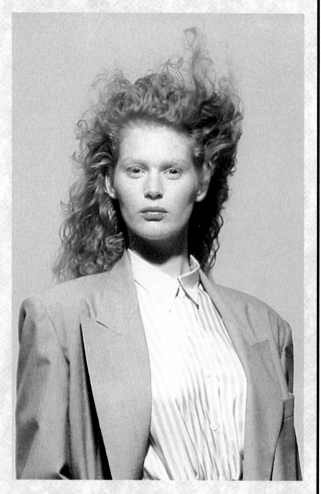

Red-heads have fewer than the average number of follicles per square centimetre of their scalp

Hairs are important sense organs, particularly those on the eyelids and eyebrows, since they are involved in the sensation of touch. It has also been suggested that hairs carry an individual's scent, by which he or she may be recognised and which may attract possible mates. Human hair almost certainly fulfils the same display functions as that of other animals.

Humans have much less visible hair than do other primates like apes and monkeys. Surprisingly, however, a square centimetre of human skin carries a greater number of hair-producing sites (called **follicles**) than the same area of the skin of other primates. We have lost the requirement for insulating our bodies, and presumably the hair which animals need for this.

Managing our hair

The appearance of the hair is the one feature of the body over which humans, unlike other primates, can have direct control. You can change the length, shape, colour and style of your hair (including, for men, facial hair) according to the age you wish to appear, and the economic and social status you want to claim.

The style, length and condition of hair all play a part in how we perceive the people we meet.

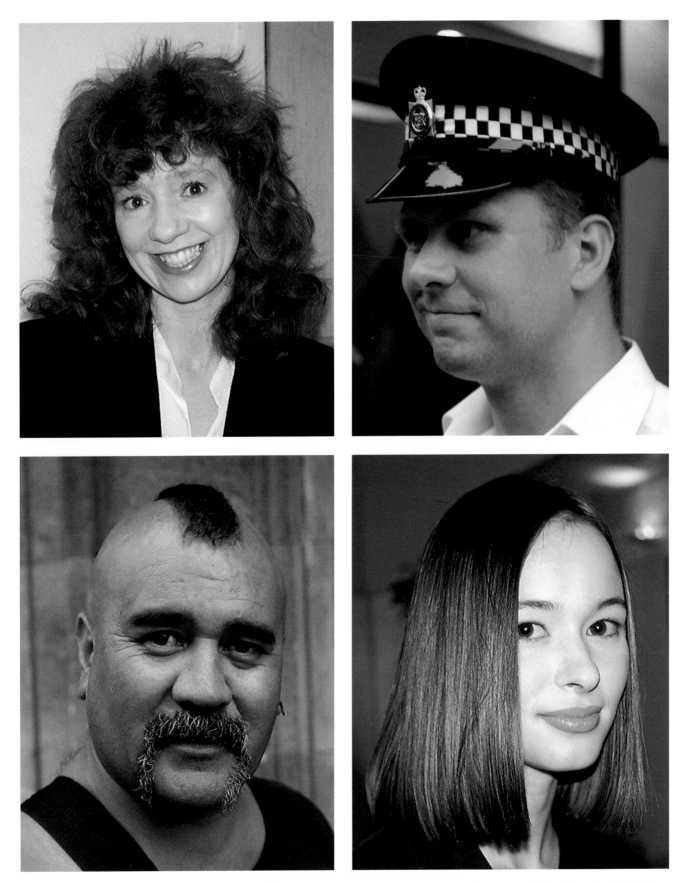

How four people – a businesswoman, a policeman, a biker and a model – have expressed their personalities through their hair

Variations in human hair

Human hair varies enormously. Different people have hair that differs in colour, in length, in diameter, and in its distribution on the body. As we shall see later, some of these factors are influenced by the person's racial type, and some by his or her age.

Types of hair

Three types of hair grow on the human body.

Lanugo hair

This is the hair that develops on an unborn baby. It begins to grow about three months after the baby's conception. The hairs are fine and soft, and they grow all over the baby's body. They all grow at the same rate, so the hairs are the same length.

Some prematurely born babies are still covered with these downy hairs. Normally they are shed about four weeks before the baby is due to be born.

Vellus hairs

Vellus hairs are short hairs, only a centimetre or two long, and contain little or no pigment. The follicles that produce them do not have grease glands (often called sebaceous glands), and never produce any other kind of hairs.

Terminal hairs

Terminal hairs are the long hairs that grow on the head and in many people on the body, arms and legs too. They are produced by follicles with sebaceous glands. In people who have inherited a tendency to baldness the hairs in these follicles gradually become thinner and shorter until they look like vellus hairs.

Variation with age

Childhood

A newly born full-term baby has two types of hair. Terminal hairs grow on the scalp and eyebrows, but nowhere else. All the rest of the hair is vellus hair.

As the baby grows, the hair on the head grows too. There are two periods during which hair grows rapidly on the scalp. In both, the hair growth begins at the forehead and then extends to the back of the neck. When the baby is two or three months old, the first hairs may be shed naturally over an area on the back of the head. This is often mistakenly thought to be due to head rubbing; hairs broken by rubbing may, however, be found on other parts of the head as well.

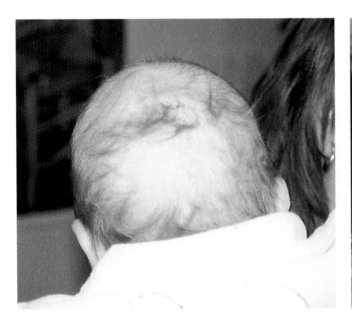

Naturally occurring hair loss, which begins at age 8–12 weeks

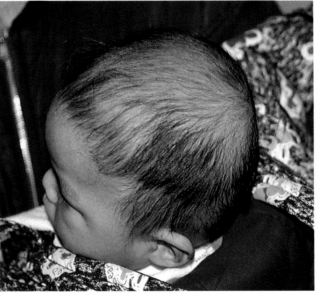

Mosaic patterns starting to develop; the beginning of hair streams can also be seen

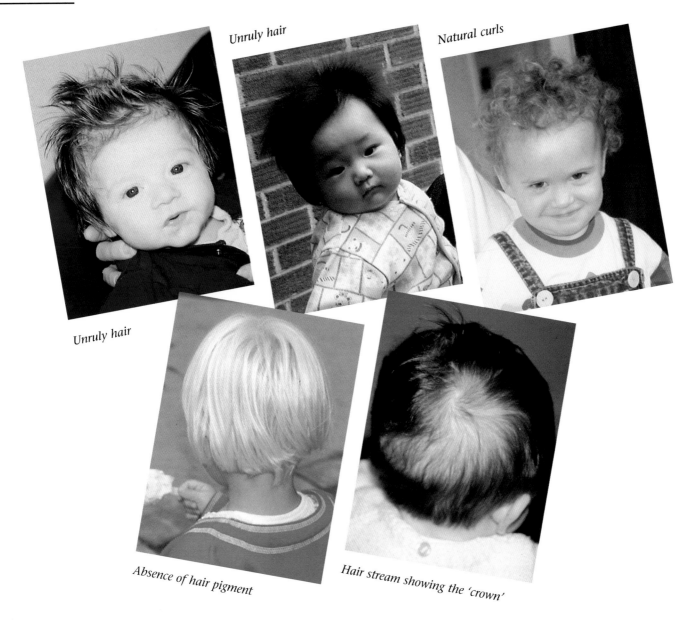

Unruly hair

Natural curls

Unruly hair

Absence of hair pigment

Hair stream showing the 'crown'

During the first year of the baby's life, all the hairs on the head grow at the same rate. At that time the head carries an even covering of hair. Then the individual hairs begin to grow independently, at different rates and in different cycles (you will read about hair growth cycles later in this chapter). Growth patterns called 'mosaics' develop.

Many children's hair shows features which are lost in adulthood. These include:

■ unruly hair which sticks straight up

■ natural curls

■ hair without pigment, which darkens as the child grows.

Adolescence

Before puberty, the scalp carries a mixture of short vellus-like hairs and longer terminal hairs, together with various 'in-between' hairs. After puberty, in both sexes, most of the scalp hairs are terminal hairs. These hairs are thicker in diameter than the childhood hairs, especially in dark-haired people.

At puberty, terminal hairs begin to appear in the armpits, groins and legs, and also (in males) on the chin, chest and forearms. How much body hair you develop is genetically determined (that is, it is inherited from your parents).

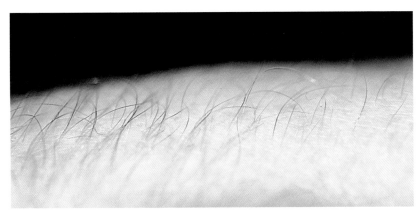

It can sometimes be difficult to distinguish between vellus and terminal hairs. (Left) These are terminal (dark) hairs growing on the forearm

(Right) Fine vellus hairs on the body

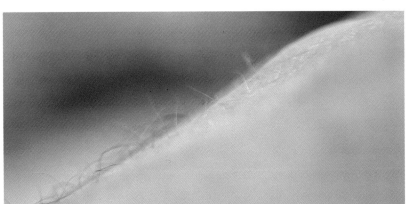

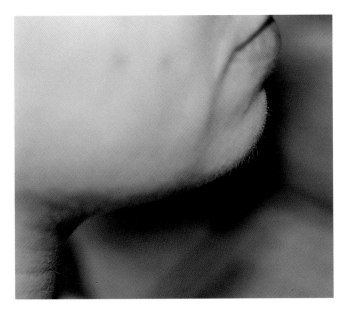

Vellus hairs on a woman's chin. These are normal: in old age, when female hormones decline, hairs on the chin can grow as strongly as terminal hairs

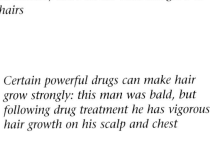

Certain powerful drugs can make hair grow strongly: this man was bald, but following drug treatment he has vigorous hair growth on his scalp and chest

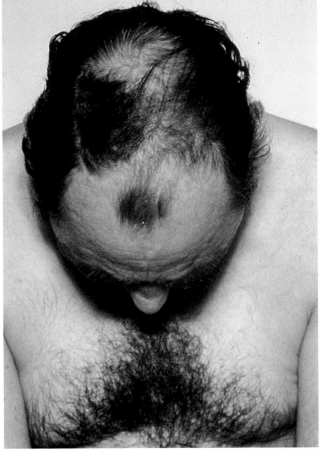

Body hair is more prominent in some races than others. In some families there is a hereditary tendency to have unusually heavy growth of facial and body hair.

Middle age and beyond

Many older people find that their hair continues to grow strongly, and that they have as much hair at 80 as they had at 50. Other people find that their hair gets thinner as they age, and that by the time they are in their 80s only a few wisps remain. Again, this is determined genetically, not by anything they have done to their hair.

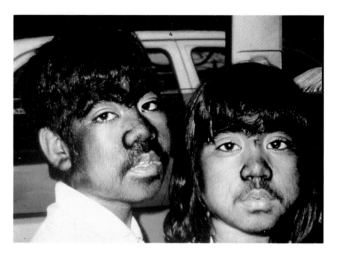

A family with a tendency to excessive hair growth

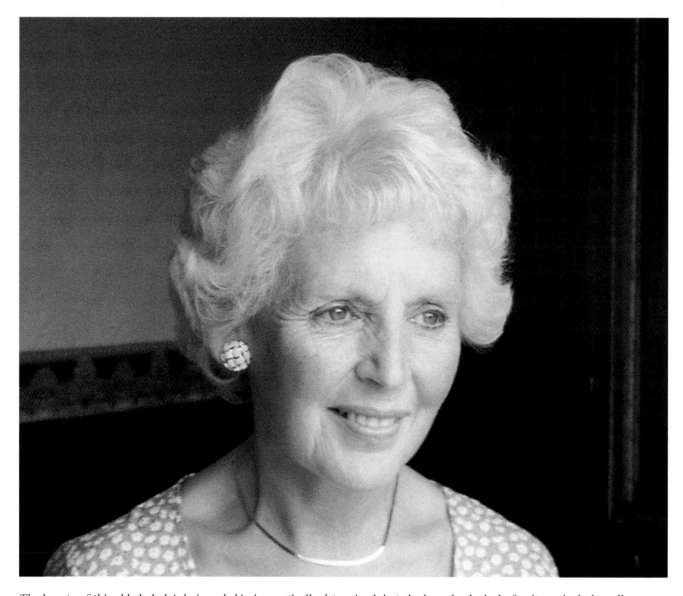

The beauty of this elderly lady's hair and skin is genetically determined, but she has also looked after it particularly well

Hair structure

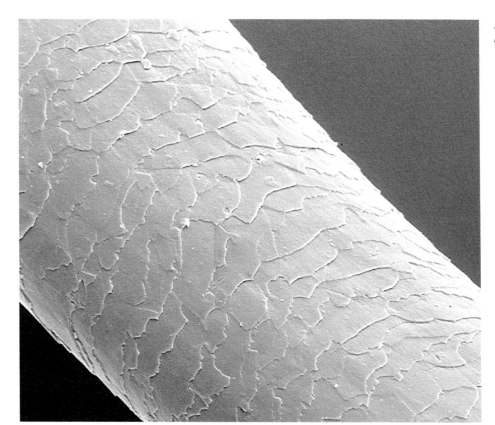

A perfect hair seen under the electron microscope

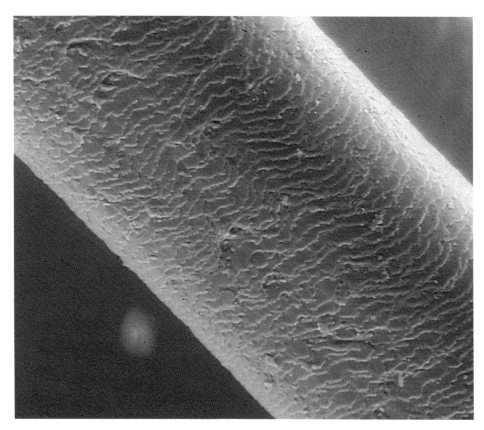

Another normal hair – but this came from one of our nearest relatives, an orang-utan!

Hair structure

In this section we look at what hair is made of, how it is able to grow as long as it does, and what helps it to grow.

A hair is a specialised outgrowth of part of the skin called the **epidermis**. It has two distinct parts, the **hair follicle** and the **hair shaft**.

The hair follicle

A hair follicle is a tiny cup-shaped pit buried deep in the fat of the scalp. The follicle is the point from which the hair grows. It is well supplied with minute blood vessels, and the blood passing through them nourishes the growing region. The temperature around the follicle is normal body temperature, and is not affected by cold or hot weather.

The hair of an animal like a cat or a horse grows at different rates depending on the

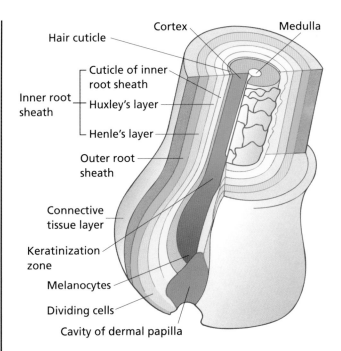

The structure of the hair bulb

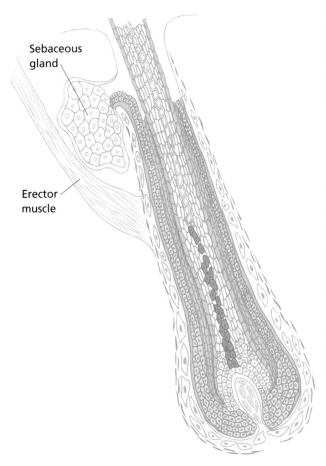

Structure of hair follicle while it is in the growing phase [Source Color Atlas of Differential Diagnosis of Hair Loss, *David A. Whiting and F. Lester Howsden, Fairfield, NJ: Canfield Publishing Inc.]*

amount of natural light, which varies according to the time of year: it grows more quickly in winter when the days are short. Human hair probably behaves in the same way, growing a little faster in winter than in summer.

The hair follicle can be divided into two regions.

The hair bulb

The hair bulb lies inside the hair follicle. It is a structure of actively growing cells, which eventually produce the long fine cylinder of a hair.

New cells are continuously produced in the lower part of the bulb. As they grow and develop they steadily push the previously formed cells upwards. When the cells reach the upper part of the bulb they begin to change, and they arrange themselves into six cylindrical layers, one inside the other. The inner three layers of cells become the actual hair. The outer three layers become the lining of the hair follicle – the inner root sheath.

Special cells in the hair bulb produce the pigment that colours the hair. The pigment is called **melanin**, and these cells are known as **melanocytes**. As the developing hair moves upwards in the follicle the melanin is carried upwards in the inner part of the hair.

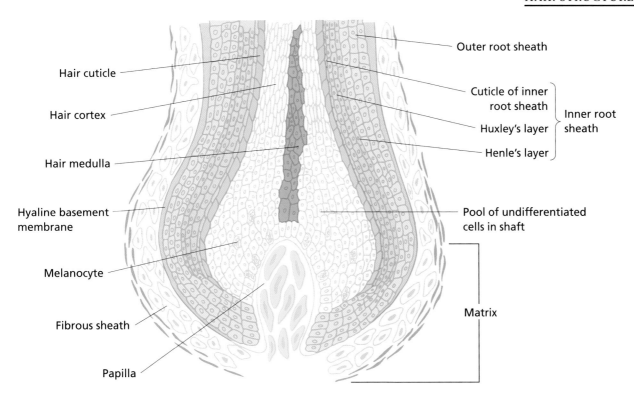

The structure of the hair bulb: the living cells gradually die, and are compressed to form the hair shaft [Source Color Atlas of Differential Diagnosis of Hair Loss, David A. Whiting and F. Lester Howsden, Fairfield, NJ: Canfield Publishing Inc.]

The mid-follicle region

In this part of the follicle the actively growing cells die and harden into what we call a hair. As the cells below continue to divide and push upwards, the hair grows upwards too, out of the skin. It now consists of a mixture of different forms of the special hair protein, **keratin**.

Some of these keratins contain a high level of sulphur, some much less. The sulphur plays an important part in the way the hair behaves, especially when it is given cosmetic treatments. You will find more about this later in the book.

The hair shaft

This is the part of the hair that can be seen above the scalp. It consists mainly of dead cells that have turned into keratins and binding material, together with small amounts of water.

Terminal hairs on the head are lubricated by a natural oil (**sebum**) produced by the sebaceous glands of the follicles. How much natural oil your glands produce is mostly determined by your genetic inheritance. But in addition boys' and girls' glands tend to produce more oil when

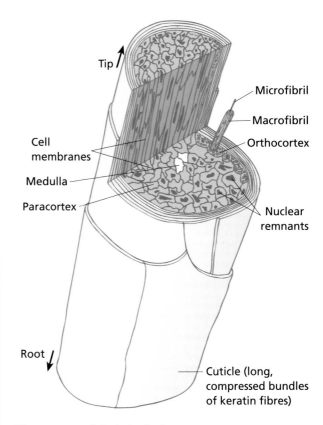

The structure of the hair shaft

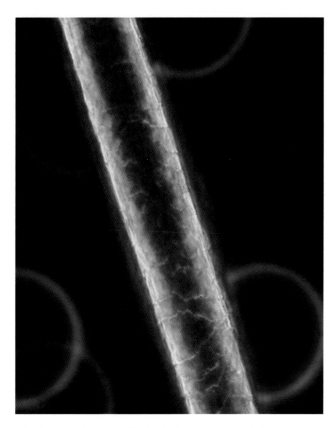

The hair shaft seen with the light microscope: light is reflected from the colourless cuticle and bent as it passes through the hair – this effect gives hair the colour we see

levels of their hormones (androgens) are high. In many teenagers, a massive surge in hormone levels leads to raised grease production. This results in a tendency to greasy hair, which many young people know all too well. The good news is that most of them outgrow it.

Structure of the hair shaft
Your smooth, glossy hairs have a more complicated structure than you might think. Each one can be compared to a tree: all its moisture lies in its centre, behind a tough outer layer of protective bark. If the 'bark' of the hair is well looked after the whole hair remains in good condition. If the 'bark' is stripped off to expose the centre the hair may break.

The centre part of the hair, called the **cortex**, makes up most of the hair shaft. It is the cortex that gives hair its special qualities such as elasticity and curl. The cortex is packed with strands of keratin, lying along the length of the hair. These keratin fibres are made of the low-sulphur keratins, and are compressed into bundles of larger fibres. These are held together by a mass of sulphur-rich keratins, the **matrix**. The fibre–matrix combination is extremely strong and resists stretching and other strains such as twisting, much as does the glass fibre–resin mixture from which many boats are built.

The cortex also contains granules of the hair pigment melanin, produced when the hair was growing in its follicle. The granules are of two types: smooth, dark granules which tend to be regularly positioned within the cortex, and lighter granules that are more irregular in shape and which are scattered randomly through the cortex. A hair may contain just one type of granule or a mixture (see also pages 16 and 59).

In some of the terminal hairs, especially grey (unpigmented) ones, the cortex has a central hollow core, the **medulla**. There are medullae in the hairs of many animals, and they play a part in the regulation of body temperature. It may be that the presence of this air space in some human hairs is an evolutionary 'throw-back' to a time when our ancestors needed extra heat insulation.

The outer layer of the hair (the 'bark') is called the **cuticle**. It is made up of between six and ten overlapping layers of long cells. Each of these cells or scales is about 0.3 micrometres thick and around 100 micrometres long, and about 10 micrometres across. (1 micrometre,

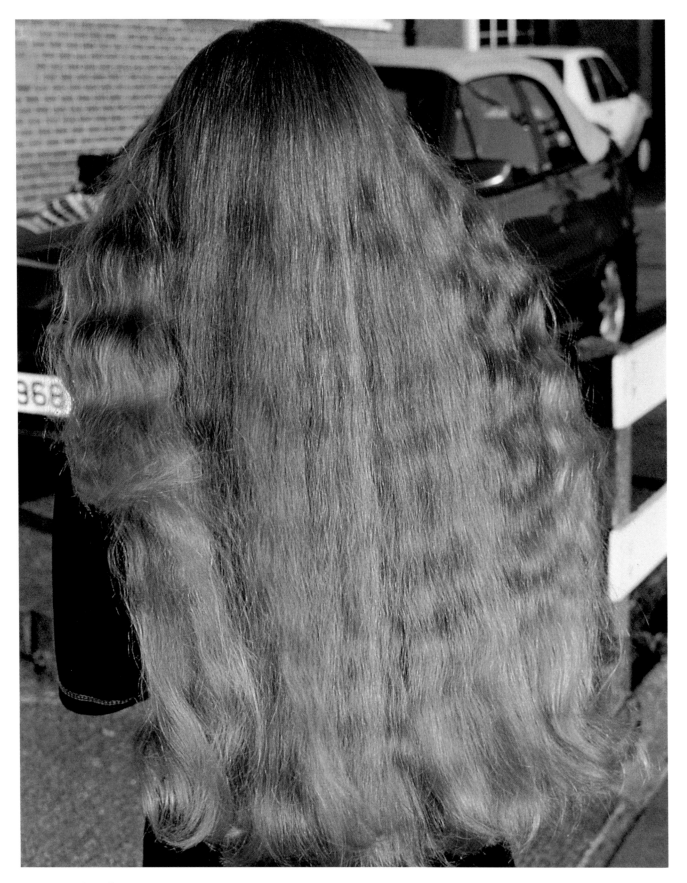

Hair in good condition

HAIR SHAFT

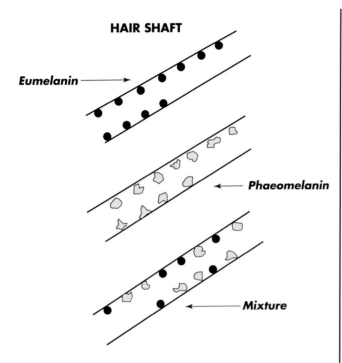

Eumelanin

Phaeomelanin

Mixture

Pigment granules in the hair shaft

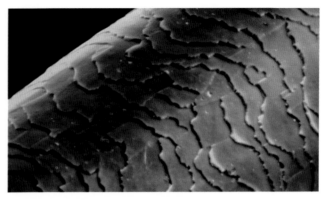

Slight lifting of the edges of the cuticles

written 1 µm, is one-millionth part of a metre = one-thousandth part of a millimetre.) The scales lie along the surface of the hair like tiles on a roof, with their free edges directed towards the tip. They cover the hair surface all the way along its length.

If you could look at a hair under a powerful microscope you would see that the scales growing over the youngest part of the hair (the part that grows closest to the scalp) are smooth and unbroken. Further along the hair, you would be able to see that they may have been damaged by cosmetic treatments and by mis-treatment such as over-energetic brushing. Little

by little they may break away, a process called **weathering** (see Chapter 2).

A healthy cuticle is more than just a protective layer. Much of the shine that makes healthy hair so attractive is due to the cuticle. Intact cuticle cells are smooth and glossy, and reflect light from their surfaces. This, together with the pigment within the cortex, gives hair its characteristic appearance.

Black hair reflects less light than blond hair does. Black hair *appears* glossier, however, because the bright bands of reflected light contrast more sharply with the darkness of the rest of the hair, as in the photograph below.

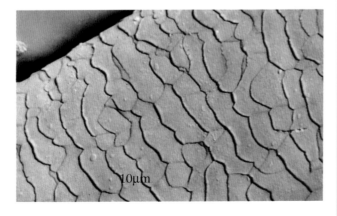

The cuticle scales on a normal hair (electronmicrograph)

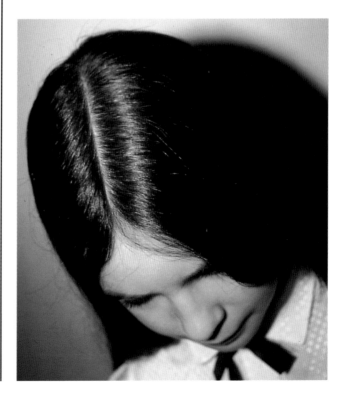

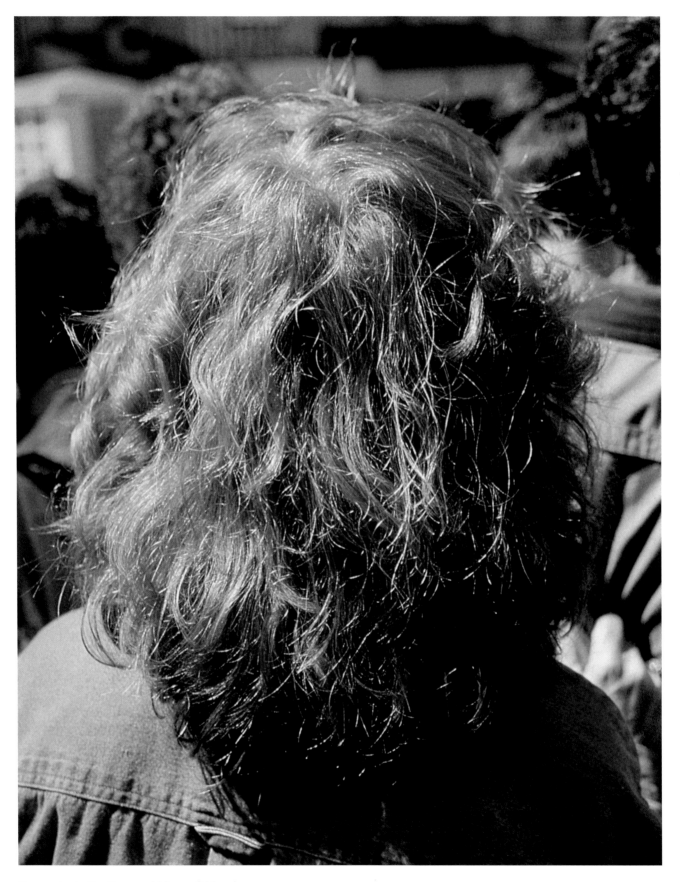

Some expert attention would be useful here!

Hair strength

Hair is surprisingly strong: a single hair can support a load of about 100 grams without breaking. You could even spin rope out of hair!

The keratin protein of the cortex is responsible for this unusual strength. The long keratin molecules in the cortex are compressed to form a regular structure, which is not only strong but also flexible.

We saw earlier that proteins are made up of long chains of amino acids. Each chain takes up a helical or coiled form, rather like a long spring, or the cable of a telephone handset.

Most protein chains are made up of various mixtures of the same 20 or so amino acids. Keratin is unique in that its chains contain high concentrations of a particular amino acid called **cystine**. The proteins in the matrix of the hair contain the highest levels of cystine.

Every cystine unit contains two **cysteine** amino acids in different chains which have come to lie near to each other and are linked together by two sulphur atoms, forming a very strong chemical bond known as a **disulphide linkage**. Many disulphide bonds form down the length of the keratin chains, joining them together like the rungs of a ladder.

The disulphide bond is one of the strongest bonds known anywhere in nature. This **cross-linking** by disulphide linkages between the keratin chains accounts for much of the strength of hair.

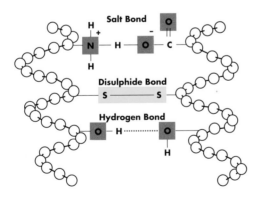

Chemical bonds within the hair maintain its shape

How hair gets its shape

The shape of a hair depends on several factors, including the shape of the hair follicle and its opening; these vary from one person to another and also between races. As keratin is hardening it is compressed into the shape of the hair follicle. The hair is then held in shape by the pattern of the chemical bonds within it. Of these, the disulphide bonds are the strongest. They can only be changed by chemical methods such as perming or relaxing.

But within each hair the keratin chains are also linked by bonds of a different kind, called **hydrogen bonds**. There are far more hydrogen bonds than disulphide linkages. The hydrogen bonds are much weaker than the disulphide linkages and more easily broken, and they give hair its flexibility. Hydrogen bonds are broken apart whenever the hair is wetted, and form again as it dries. When they break the shape of the hair changes. If the wet hair is then wound on to rollers it will form a new shape, and if it is dried on the rollers it will keep this shape.

This is the basis of the **setting** process. The change in shape is only temporary. It is lost when the hair is dampened, because the new hydrogen bonds are broken again.

Hair dimensions

People describe their hair as being thick or thin, coarse or fine. What they are usually talking about is the amount of coverage their hair gives to the head. This coverage depends on two things: how many hairs there are, and the thickness (diameter) of each hair shaft.

People vary a lot in how many hairs they have, and also in how closely together they grow. The 'average' person has around 100,000 hairs, but people with very dense hair may have as many as 150,000.

The diameter of the hair shaft varies too. It is usually around 57–90 μm in Europeans. This is much less than in Asians, in whom it can be 120 μm. (These are general figures, representing a wide range of values.)

Hair that is both dense and thick looks completely different from that of someone who has fewer and finer hairs.

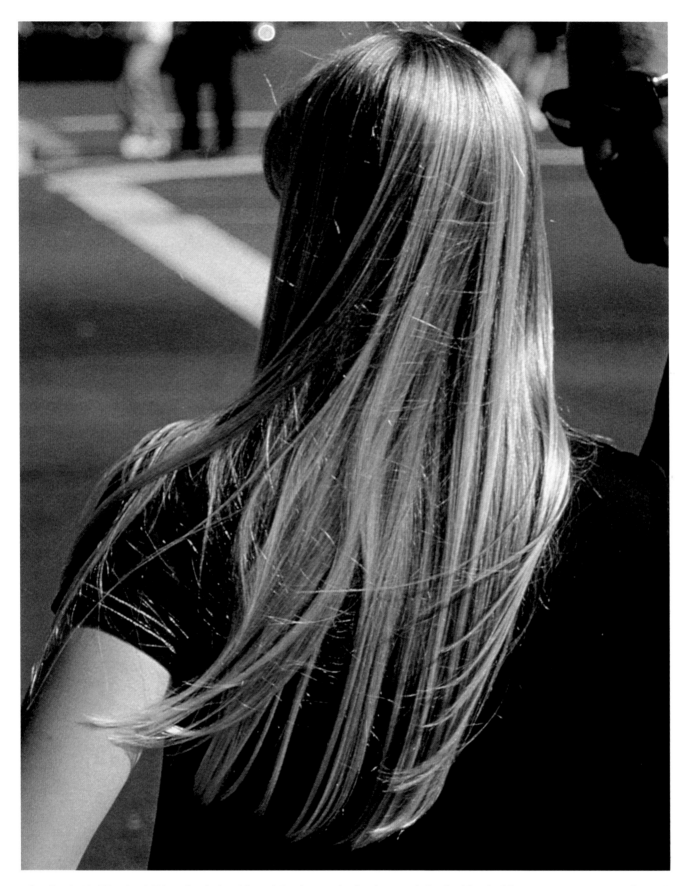

The classic 'California girl' has fine hair with mainly phaeomelanin pigment (it is also bleached by constant exposure to the sun)

The hair growth cycle

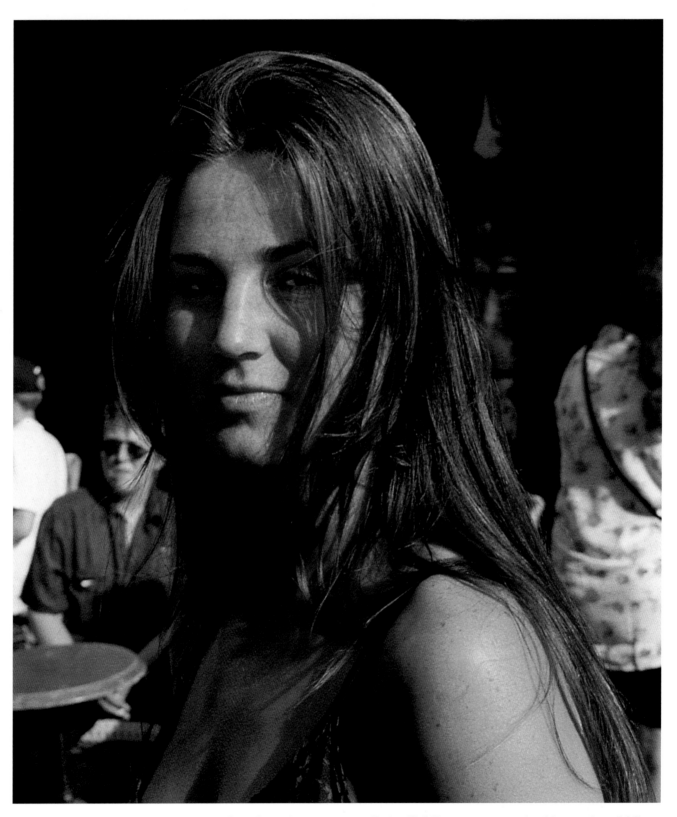

Each of these long hairs has been growing for at least six years: eventually it will fall out spontaneously; this growth and fall makes up the hair cycle

The hair growth cycle

Each individual hair is formed inside a hair bulb deep in a hair follicle. The follicle is a tiny but powerful factory, which throughout many people's lifetime hardly ever stops working. From a baby's birth for many decades, as much as a century in some people, the follicle continues to produce hairs. Each hair grows for many years: during this time it will be shampooed, conditioned, cut, blown dry, exposed to sun and wind, coloured or bleached or permed. None of these treatments affects the growth of the hair in the hair bulb, even though some may seriously damage the hair shaft. Finally the hair spontaneously falls out. The follicle rests for a little while, and then starts to produce yet another new hair. This is the **hair cycle**.

You need to know about the hair cycle in order to understand many of the problems people have with their hair. These can range from the sudden appearance of hairless patches to complete baldness in men, and sometimes in women too.

Stages of the hair cycle

Between starting to grow and falling out years later, each hair passes through three distinct stages. These are so important that they have been given special names: **anagen** (the growing phase), **catagen** (the intermediate phase) and **telogen** (the shedding phase).

We shall look at these three stages in turn.

Anagen (the growing phase)

The **anagen** phase of a new hair starts at the moment it begins to grow. At that time there is very active growth in the hair bulb. This usually

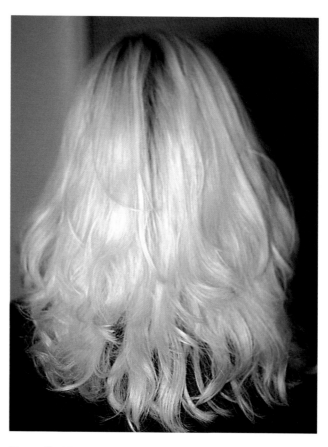

Naturally blond hair: this lady's anagen phase lasts for about four years

---

HAIR FACTS

The phases of the hair growth cycle

It is easy to remember the lengths of the different phases of the growth cycle. Very roughly speaking:

anagen	1000 days (or more)
catagen	10 days
telogen	100 days

The hair growth cycle, showing the changes from the growing of a new hair (anagen) to its shedding (telogen): notice how in anagen the hair bulb lies deep inside the scalp and then rises towards the surface before the hair is shed, then moves down again as the new hair grows

Anagen ⟶ Catagen ⟶ Telogen ⟶ Anagen ⟶

Old club hair

Hair matrix
Club hair
Hair papilla
Epithelial column

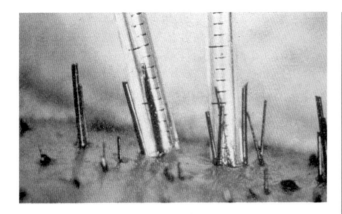

A method of measuring the rate of hair growth: both cut hairs and newly emerging hairs can be seen

lasts for some years, generally between three and seven, without interruption. Since human hairs grow at a rate of roughly 1 centimetre a month, hairs can grow to a length of a metre or so.

As we have seen, hair may grow more quickly in winter than in summer. Hair growth varies with the season as a result of a change in the difference between hair follicles in the growing and shedding phases.

Pigment (melanin) is made in the hair bulb throughout this phase of the hair cycle. Less pigment is made in the hair of older people. This is why white hairs start to appear, even though the hair itself may still be growing strongly.

In some older people the hair cycle becomes shorter, the follicles gradually give up producing long, strong hair, and the hairs become thinner and shorter. The result may be a general thinning of the hair, or even a degree of baldness.

HAIR FACTS

Follicle activity

In everyday life, nothing interrupts the activity of the hair follicle. Nothing that is put on the scalp or hair can interfere with the growth of the hairs. Only severe burns or scars can affect the hair follicle.

Certain drugs that are given for cancer treatment can prevent hairs from growing. (This is discussed later in this chapter.) Almost always, however, the interruption is only temporary and hairs begin to grow again when the medication is stopped.

Catagen (the intermediate phase)

The anagen phase is followed by a short resting phase. This **catagen** phase lasts for between two and four weeks in the human scalp. No pigment is made during that time, and the follicle stops producing hair. The base of the follicle moves upwards towards the surface of the skin.

Telogen (the shedding phase)

The **telogen** phase lasts for three or four months. This is the time at which a new hair begins to grow from the hair follicle. As it grows upwards the old hair will be shed naturally or may be pulled out, which happens easily and painlessly with telogen hairs. These are the hairs that come out when you shampoo or brush your hair.

Shedding is part of the normal process of the replacement of old hair with new. At any one time, around one in ten of the follicles on an individual's head are in the shedding phase.

The new hair emerges from the same opening at the surface of the skin as the old one, and the hair cycle begins again.

Hair length

How long anagen lasts is determined genetically, and varies between the sexes and from one person to another. It is the length of this time that decides how long the hair will

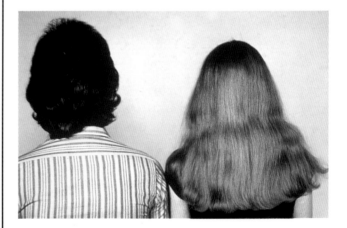

Differences in hair length depend on the length of anagen, which is genetically determined. These two people started off with hair of the same length and went without a haircut for 18 months: the man's hair grows only to his collar before it falls out naturally, but the woman's anagen period is clearly much longer [reproduced from Diseases of the Hair and Scalp, *A. Rook and R. Dawber (eds), 2nd edn, Oxford: Blackwell Scientific Publications, 1981]*

HAIR FACTS

The growth of human hair

- Each human head carries roughly 100,000 hair follicles.

- Each follicle can grow many hairs over a lifetime: on average, each grows a new hair around twenty times.

- Not all these follicles are actively growing hairs at any one time. From the moment when it is first formed, each follicle undergoes repeated cycles of active growth and rest. The length of the cycle varies with the individual, and also with the part of the body on which the hair is growing.

- The hairs on an adult scalp do not grow in unison, as they do in an unborn baby. They are 'out of cycle' with each other. If this were not so, everyone would go temporarily bald from time to time.

- The growing and shedding of hair as a whole seems to happen at random, but for each hair follicle the process is precisely controlled. No one knows for certain, however, exactly how the body controls these cycles.

- Plucking a hair from a follicle brings forward the next period of hair growth in that follicle.

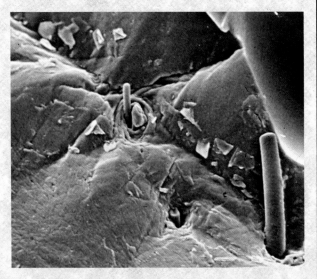

Electronmicrograph showing new hairs emerging from the hair follicles of the scalp

- Over the years, the number of follicles capable of growing hair declines naturally. The decline is especially noticeable on the top of the head. Some follicles increasingly produce only fine, short non-pigmented hairs that look more like vellus hairs than terminal hairs. In older women, this leads to a general thinning of hair. In men it tends to lead to common baldness. If you look at a bald scalp you will see these fine, poorly pigmented hairs.

---

grow before it falls out. Anagen lasts between three and seven years in most people.

- As we have seen, a hair grows at a rate of about 1 centimetre a month.

- After one year it will be 12 cm long. After five years it will be 60 cm long.

- Waist-length hair is 80–90 cm long, and will have taken about seven years to grow.

- Shoulder-length hair will have taken only about three years. Thus only people with long anagen times can expect to grow their hair down to the waist.

As people grow older the period of anagen shortens. For example, the hair of someone with a five-year anagen can grow to a length of 60 cm before it enters the shedding phase. If their anagen period drops to three years as they age, their hair will then grow only to shoulder length before it falls out or is brushed out.

So when a scanty-haired elderly lady boasts that when she was a girl she could sit on her hair, she may very well be telling you the truth!

What controls hair growth?

No one can answer this question with certainty. What we *do* know is that it takes a lot to stop hair growing!

General health and nutritional factors are increasingly believed to be important for healthy hair growth. We do know that serious anaemia affects hair growth. So too does starvation: people who go on a crash diet may start to lose their hair some six to ten weeks later. Many alcoholics have poor hair growth or even hair loss because their way of life tends to lead to malnutrition.

Some minerals may be particularly important for hair growth. For example, some people who lack zinc in their diet produce only fine, sparse hairs and even lose their hair. Vitamin B, also known as panthenol, plays a part in hair growth. It also improves the physical properties (elasticity, strength and gloss) of the hair shaft.

The hair cycle for each individual hair is influenced by the levels of various hormones in the blood. Thyroid hormone speeds up growth in resting hair follicles. Steroids taken by mouth slow it down, though steroids inhaled for the treatment of asthma do not affect hair growth.

The hair of the scalp is, however, most sensitive to the effects of male hormones (**androgens**), which are in the blood of people of both sexes (only in different proportions in men and women). Androgens are the most important factor regulating hair growth, and also the thickness of the hair shaft. Female hormones (**oestrogens**), which both sexes have too, slow down hair growth during the growing period but also make that period longer. Many women notice a difference in their hair growth during pregnancy. At this time women have vast amounts of oestrogen in their blood, far outweighing their male hormones. It is the balance between the male and female hormones which decides the growth of the hair.

We have already seen how at puberty the immature vellus-like hairs on our bodies can change to terminal hairs. This change results from the dramatic rise in androgen levels at that time. It is especially noticeable in young men. Young women who suffer from the condition of anorexia nervosa, however, stop having periods and produce very little oestrogen: their natural androgens tend to thicken their fine vellus-like hairs in the same way.

The effects of androgens continue long after puberty. Some areas of the skin respond to these hormones more vigorously than others do, and at different times of life. Pubic and armpit hair begins to grow at or soon after puberty. Most men's beards do not grow strongly until the owners reach their thirties. The growth of chest hair reaches a peak even later, and hair in the nose and ears grows most in late middle age.

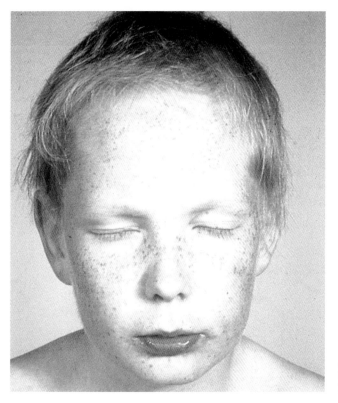 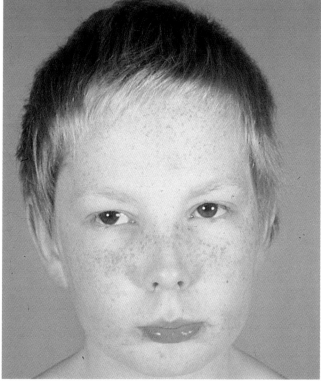

(Left) This boy has a zinc deficiency, and his hair is very thin and sparse; (right) after treatment his hair is growing more strongly

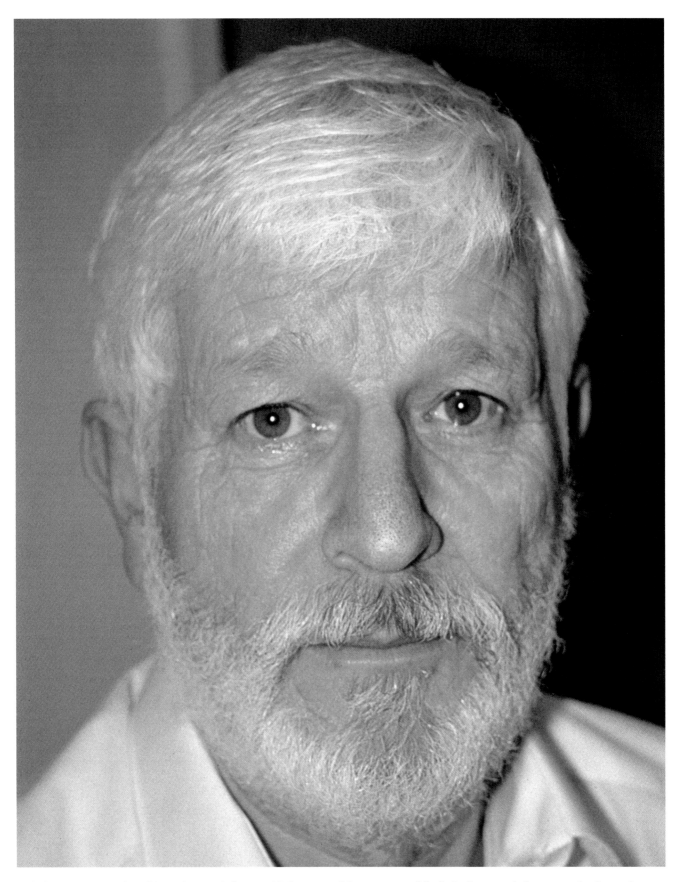

A full set: growing a beard is easier at 50 than at 15, because of the response of the hair site to male hormones (androgens)

Hair patterns

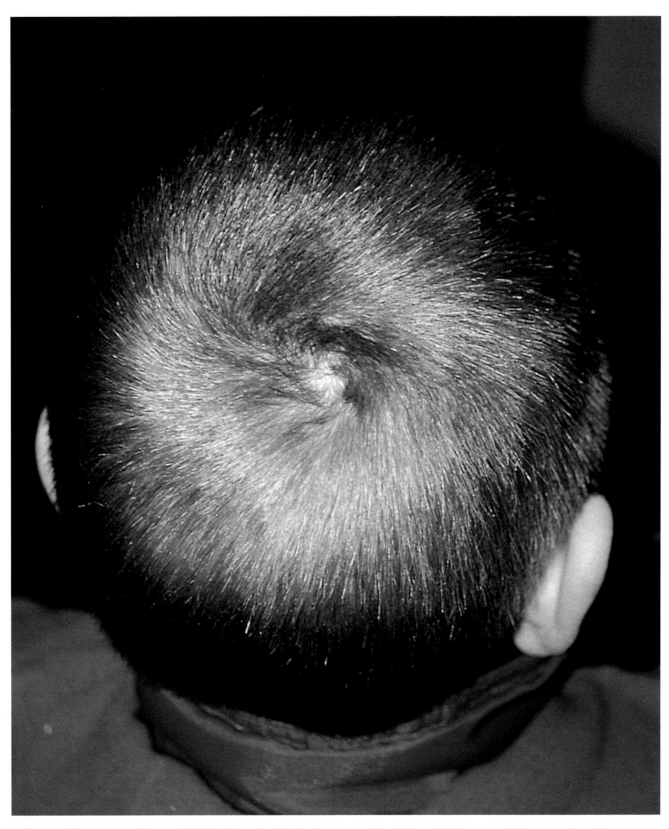

Hair grows in patterns or 'streams': this is the typical clockwise stream. Knowledge of hair streams is important in styling

HAIR FACTS

Effects of damage on hair growth

Damage to the skin starts up a new growing phase in resting follicles. Wounds cause hair growth in the skin around them, provided there is no scarring in the follicle.

It is not true that cutting your hair makes it grow faster or thicker. Nor does shaving your legs make the hair grow coarser – it just feels that way. The width of the hair shaft is determined by your genes, and is not affected by anything you do to your skin or to the hair shaft itself.

Effects of chemotherapy on hair patterns

Treatment of cancer with drugs may cause apparent complete hair loss. This is because these drugs are designed to kill cancer cells, which are cells that are growing out of control. Other cells that are growing very actively may be affected too: these may include cells in the bowel lining and also in hair follicles. This leads to a 'break' in growth and an inherent weakness. Once the drugs are stopped the patient's hair starts to grow back, but when it reaches the surface it tends to break. This is what causes the apparent hair loss.

The hair that subsequently grows may may look quite different from the old. This is because the growth patterns of the sensitive cells of the hair bulb may still be upset by the effects of the drug.

Hair patterns

Hair streams

A hair does not grow straight up out of the skin, but leaves the follicle at a definite and predetermined angle. This angle determines the direction along which the hair will lie, and determines the patterns or streams that the hairs make on the head. Often the streams spiral outwards from a central point (or points) on the crown of the head. Usually these spirals, or 'whorls', run in a clockwise direction.

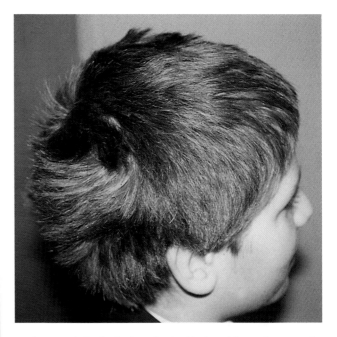

A characteristic clockwise whorl of hair, with an element of unruliness

The classical 'cowlick', seen in around 7% of children, is due to a particular hair stream on the forehead.

Unruly hair in children may be the result of scalp hair patterning. Another possible reason is an unusual structure of the hair shaft.

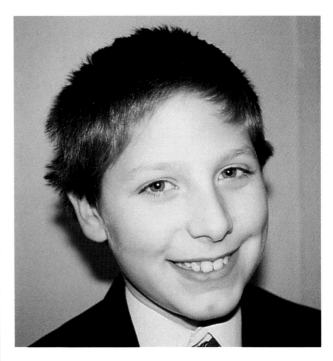

A boy with 'cowlick' hair

Hairlines

Forehead hairlines are determined genetically. The hairline that you were born with may well be the one you ultimately have in your adult life. Nearly all women keep their frontal line unchanged from childhood to old age, although some women's hairlines may seem to recede because their hair gets thinner. About half of all men may expect the hairline to recede to some extent, however.

Examining hair

From time to time doctors, scientists, hair stylists and technicians are all asked, for different reasons, to examine someone's hair. All of them need to know the right methods to use, and to understand the hair growth cycle and the cosmetic treatments and weathering processes that affect the hair's appearance.

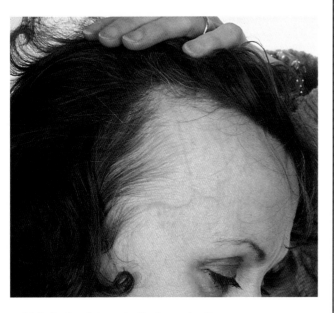

A high forehead (genetically determined)

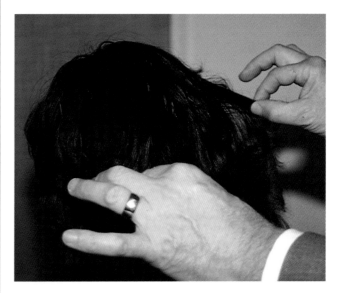

Examining hair: a gentle pull on the hair can indicate the extent to which hairs are being shed

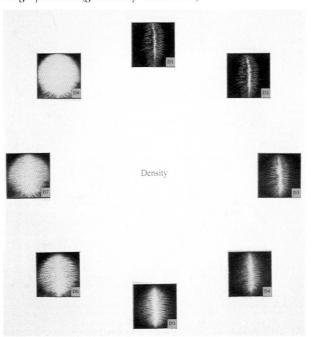

Density

The decline in density of a woman's hair through the decades: the stages numbered D5 and D6 are normal for a woman in her eighties, but would be quite abnormal for someone in her twenties or thirties [reproduced by permission of Dr. R. Dawber]

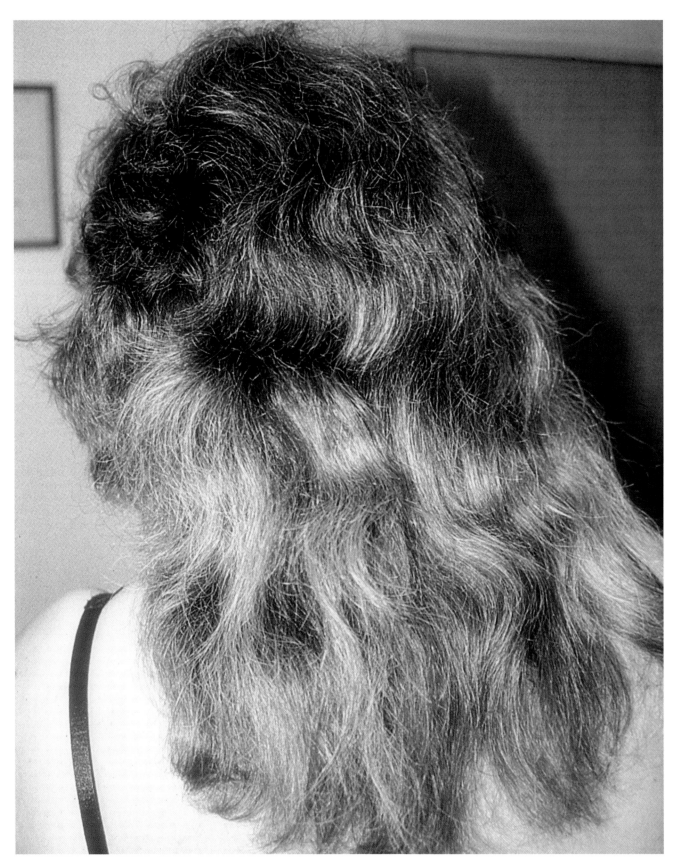

Correct examination of hair, whether in the doctor's surgery (above) or in the salon, is important in understanding its medical or cosmetic condition; this lady's hair is a challenge to the stylist if not to the doctor

Loose hairs

Many people worry because they often find loose hairs on their clothes, or after shampooing, and they become terrified in case they may lose some or most of their hair.

If you pull the hair lightly with your hand, you may well find that a few hairs do come out. These are almost certainly hairs that are ready to fall anyway – telogen hairs. You can confirm this by looking at the roots in a good light. A telogen follicle root is a little hard, white bead. Brushed-out hairs all have this kind of root.

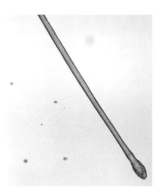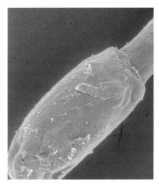

A normal telogen hair with a hard 'club' end, seen under (left) a light microscope and (right) an electron microscope

On the other hand, the root of a hair that is *pulled* out is fat, soft to the touch and sticky – it will stick to your hand, because it still carries fluid from the follicle. And pulling it out hurts! This is an anagen hair, one which was not ready to be shed.

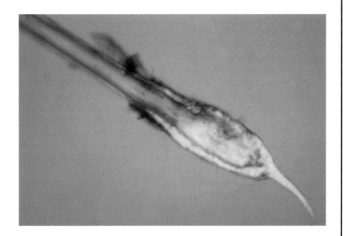

An anagen hair that has been plucked out: notice the soft, sticky tail

---

HAIR FACTS

Shampooing and hair loss

Telogen hairs fall out very easily. As catagen hairs change to telogen, the tails are slowly reabsorbed into the follicle. The roots of hairs in these early stages of telogen may be pulled out before they are quite ready to come out, especially if the hair is shampooed more energetically than usual. This is why, whenever there is a change in the shampooing or conditioning regime, or a move to new brushes, loose hairs are often found for two or three days after the change. People often blame a new shampoo or conditioner, claiming in horror, 'I put this product on my head and now I'm losing my hair'. The loose hairs are nothing to do with the product: the condition will settle down in a day or two, once these hairs have been shed.

In normal circumstances, when you find loose hair in the plug-hole after shampooing the new hair is already re-growing.

Closer examination

Hair stylists and technicians examine the whole head of hair as part of their everyday practice. Matters to note include racial type, hair length and hair thickness, and if there is evidence of weathering, of previous cosmetic treatments such as perming and tinting and of accumulated hair spray.

A closer examination of the roots under a good light usually indicates the real state of the hair. The first centimetre or two of growth may look very different from the rest. This could indicate a change in the treatment that the hair has received, perhaps to a persistently harsh regime.

Next comes a look at the individual hair shafts with the naked eye. This may not reveal much, unless there is unusually serious damage. In very long hair that has weathered, the end may look a different colour from the rest, or perhaps less glossy. This is almost certainly the onset of split ends.

Under the microscope, however, a very different picture may emerge. Hair scientists use both ordinary microscopes and electron

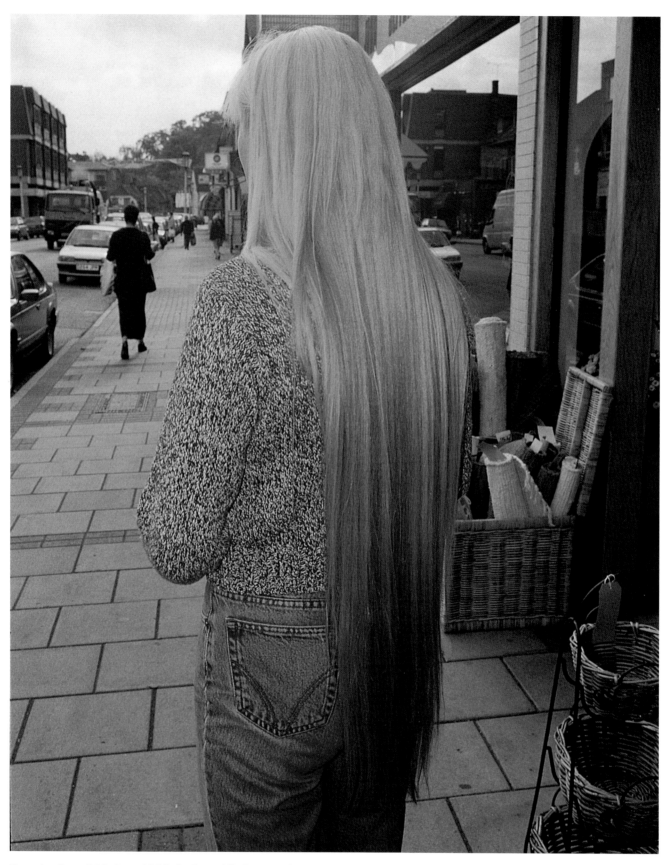

Examination of this beautiful hair showed little or no damage until the last few centimetres; this is because it has never been processed

microscopes to examine hair in the laboratory. These allow them to understand what happens to hair when it is heated, permed, tinted and so forth. You will find examples of what can be seen under both kinds of microscope throughout this book.

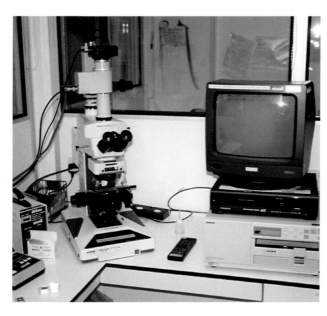

A hair scientist's laboratory: the electron microscope

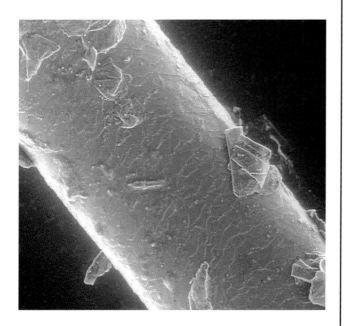

A hair, carrying some normal fragments of debris, seen under the electron microscope

The physical properties of hair

In this section we look at the ways in which hair can change or be changed. It can be stretched, bent and curled. It can absorb moisture or lose it. Its behaviour can alter when it is wetted or when it is brushed. We look at the special properties of hair, such as its elasticity, porosity and texture.

Understanding these properties is important for all of us as we cope with our hair under different circumstances. It is especially important for the hair stylist who has to decide on styles and to suggest continuing hair care regimes for clients.

Elasticity

This is one of the most important properties of hair. Because of its elasticity, hair can resist forces that could change its shape, its volume or its length. Its elasticity lets it spring back to its original form without damage.

When healthy hair is wetted and stretched, it can increase in length by up to 30% and still return to its original length when it is dried. Stretching it more than this will tend to damage it, however, leading to permanent lengthening and even breaking.

The elasticity of hair depends on the long keratin fibres in the cortex. Chemical treatments of hair such as perming and bleaching can alter the cortex after repeated damage, and change the hair's elasticity. Hair with poor elasticity will stretch only to a limited extent. It will not curl, it will break easily when it is groomed and it cannot be permed satisfactorily.

Both natural sunlight and artificial ultraviolet light break down chemicals in the hair and damage its elasticity in the same way that bleaching does, though to a much lesser degree.

A stylist must always examine the elasticity of a client's hair before deciding on any chemical procedure.

Static electricity

When dry hair is rubbed, as it is whenever it is brushed or combed, static electric charge builds up on the hairs. This is especially noticeable in hot, dry weather. The charges tend to push each other apart, and as a result charged hairs can

The physical properties of hair

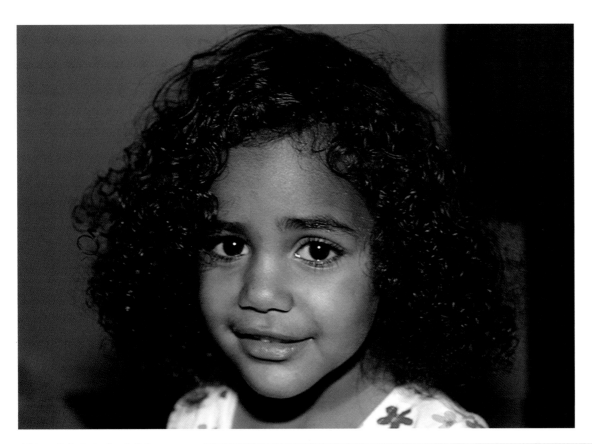

Although hair is dead, it has many characteristics that persuade us it is 'alive': twists, curls and knots are reflections of the flexibility and other inherent properties of each individual hair shaft

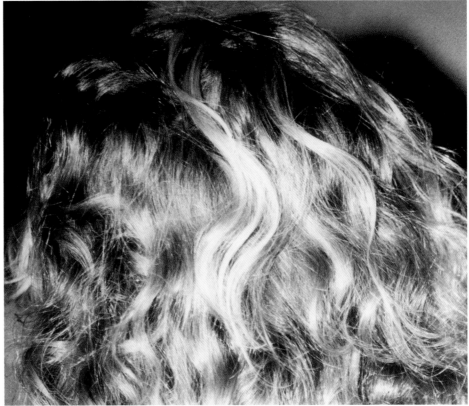

never lie smoothly against each other. The result is 'fly away' hair, which stands out from the head and looks unmanageable.

Conditioners, and shampoos with high levels of conditioning agents in them, leave the surfaces of the hair smooth. There is therefore less friction when the hairs are rubbed: hence less static electricity builds up on them, and 'fly away' is reduced.

Moisture content

The moisture content of hair is greater when the atmosphere is moist and humid, and less when the air is dry. The reason why hair 'collapses' in hot, humid atmospheres is summed up by:

heat and humidity → more moisture
                   → less static electricity
                   → collapse

In dry conditions:

heat and dryness → less moisture
                 → more static electricity
                 → more volume (body)

When hair is wet the cortex swells and the edges of the cuticle scales tend to lift. The hair surface temporarily loses its smoothness.There is therefore more friction when wet hair is rubbed than when it is dry. This is what can lead to matting and tangles developing during over-vigorous shampooing (there is *not* greater static charge on wet hair than on dry).

These tangles are one of the reasons why many children hate having their hair washed, and the problem is easy to avoid.

Hair diameter
The elastic properties of both wet and dry hair are related to the diameter of the hair shaft. The thicker the hair, the more it will tend to resist stretching.

Porosity

In a normal, undamaged hair shaft, very little water can get either into or out of the cortex. This is because the cuticle covering the cortex is intact, and is then almost (but not quite) waterproof. Shampoos do not damage the

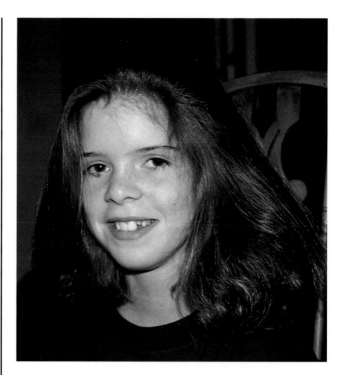

Particularly thick, strong hair: the hairs grow densely and each has a wide diameter

cuticle. When hair is permed or tinted, however, the chemicals have to penetrate the cortex in order to react with the keratin inside it. Increasing the temperature, or applying an alkaline lotion, separates the scales of the cuticle enough to allow the chemicals to pass through. After the processing is finished the scales gradually close up again.

But if hair is processed too many times the cuticle scales may never return to their original tightness and the protection they once offered is lost. The cuticle can also be damaged in the same way by too much blow drying, curling irons that are too hot, and the effects of wind and sun. The hair becomes increasingly porous, and water can then pass in and out of the cortex.

Over-porous hair is dry, and tends to develop split ends. The damaged cuticle is fragile, and the damage worsens as time goes by. The greater the damage, the more the cortex swells with water whenever the hair is washed, but the more water it loses when it dries. The repeated wetting and drying of the cortex gradually weakens the hair.

Texture

Much of the attraction of a beautiful head of hair lies in its texture, or feel. The texture of hair depends on several things.

The first is the average diameter of the individual hairs. We have seen that these vary widely. The larger the hair diameter, the coarser it will feel.

Secondly, different people's hair naturally feels different: some hard and others soft, some silky and others wiry. The reasons underlying these differences are still a matter for scientists to argue over.

Thirdly, the texture is affected by the degree of weathering of the hair.

Finally, hair texture is affected by what has been put on it. Repeated lavish applications of hair spray gives hair a different feel from that of hair that has been freshly washed and conditioned. Conditioners make hair feel soft and smooth. Conditioners that contain silicones even give a slightly different feel from those that don't (most manufacturers do put silicones into conditioners nowadays, however, as they protect the hair cuticle). Contrary to popular belief, this altered feel is *not* a sign of build-up.

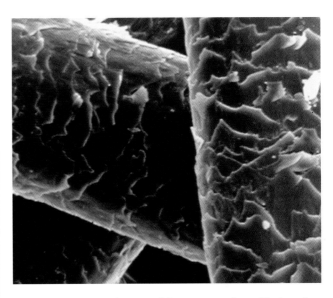

Damage to the cuticle, caused by over-perming will alter the texture of the hair

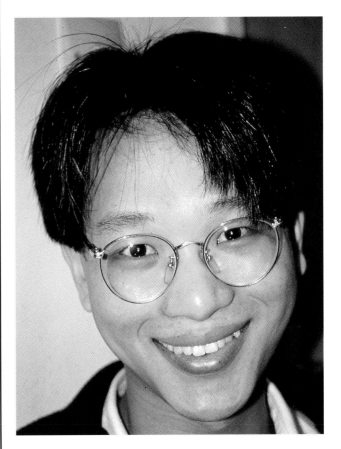

Great hair – thick and perfectly straight, with a texture like that of a horse's mane!

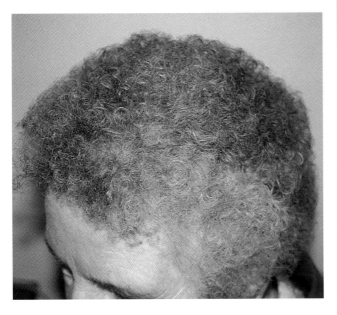

In later life this lady's hair has become naturally shorter and thinner, with less body; perming, which she has chosen as a way of correcting this, has resulted in dryness and loss of texture

Hair types

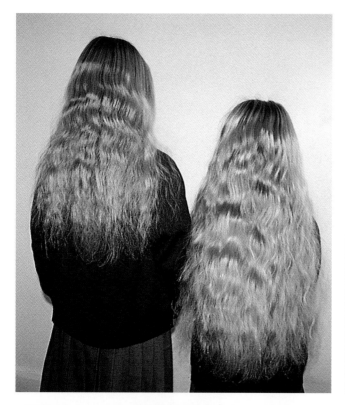

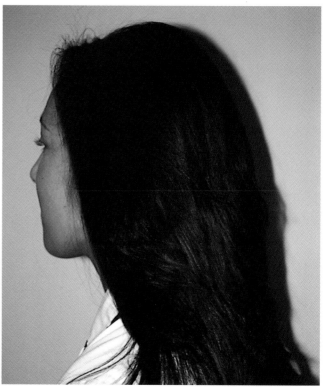

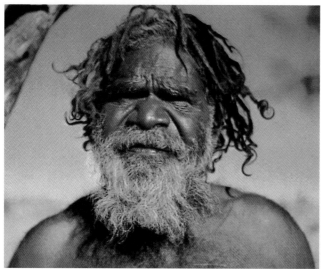

Our hair type is determined by our genes (see text): (top left) Caucasian sisters with identical hair; (top right) Mongoloid hair, straight and dense; (lower left) Australian Aborigine – scientists are uncertain of the genetic origin of his hair type, but some Indian fakirs have similar hair; (lower right) the tight woolly curls of typical Negroid hair

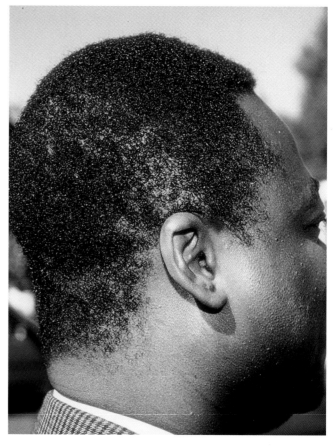

Hair types

The range of different types of hair is enormous, ranging from tight wiry curls to ruler-straight. The colour and shape of hair vary too. What accounts for these differences?

The type of hair you have is inherited from your parents. We may look back further, and say that it is determined by the part of the world in which your ancestors originated. It all depends on the race, or mixture of races, from which they came. In the very earliest days of human evolution, three basic racial groups of people seem to have existed on this planet. These spread out across the world and became mixed together. They are especially well mixed in countries where there has been massive immigration, such as the U.S.A. over the last few hundred years.

Scientists have identified three basic types of hair in today's human population, and have related them to these three early races: **Mongoloid**, **Caucasoid** and **Negroid**.

The three types of hair not only look quite different, but the differences in their responses to physical and chemical damage can be remarkable.

Mongoloid

These are people from the Orient, for example from China and Japan. Their hair is very straight, and always black in colour.

Caucasoid

The Caucasoid group is the most 'mongrel' of the three racial groups. Modern Caucasoids are very varied, even though they are descended from the same group of ancestors. They range from the fair-skinned people of north-west Europe to the widely varying peoples of the Indian subcontinent. Their hair may be either wavy or straight, and the diameter varies widely too. The colour ranges from black to a pale blond that is almost white, including just about every possible shade in between.

Negroid

Negroid people originated in Africa. Their hair is black and tightly curled. It tends to be woolly and dry, and is extremely easily damaged by heat or chemicals.

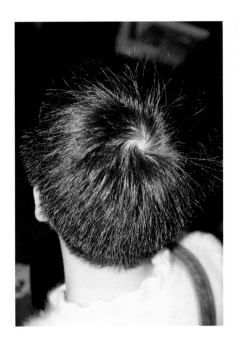

Mongoloid is straight and thick, and resists damage well

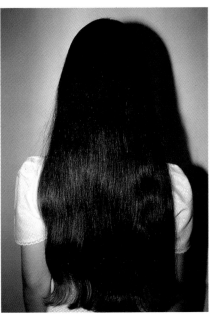

Caucasoid hair can be anything from blond to black in colour, and may be curly, wavy or straight

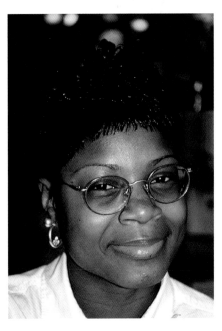

Negroid hair is vulnerable to damage, because of its shape and twisted structure

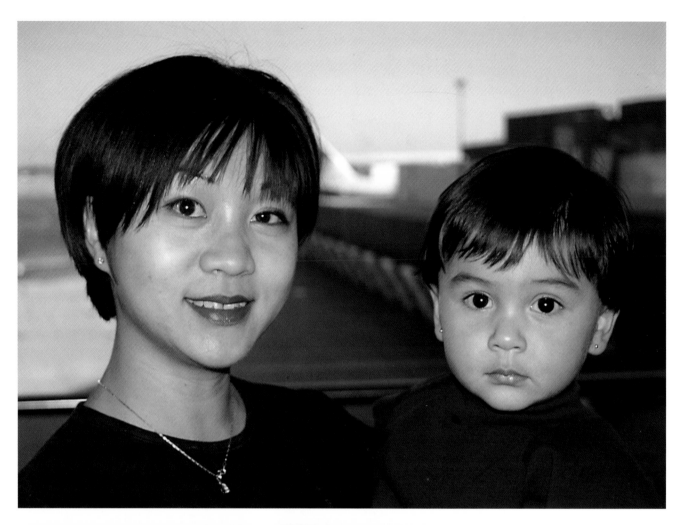

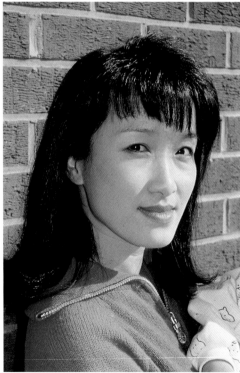

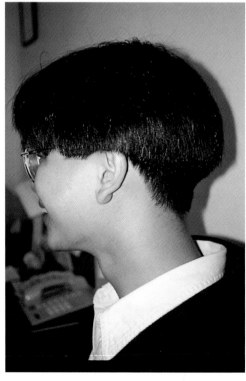

These very different people all have Mongoloid hair – thick, black and perfectly straight

*A type of Caucasoid hair that is typical
of people of Latin descent*

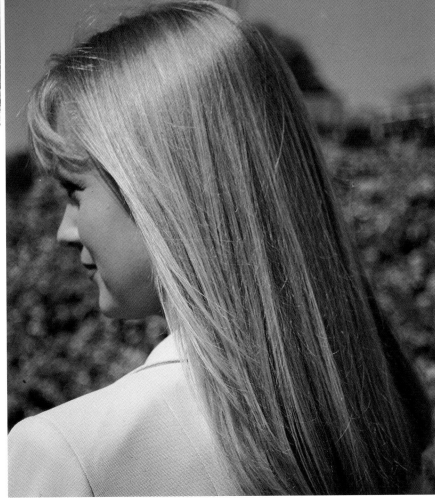

*Naturally blond Caucasoid hair,
characteristic of north-western Europe*

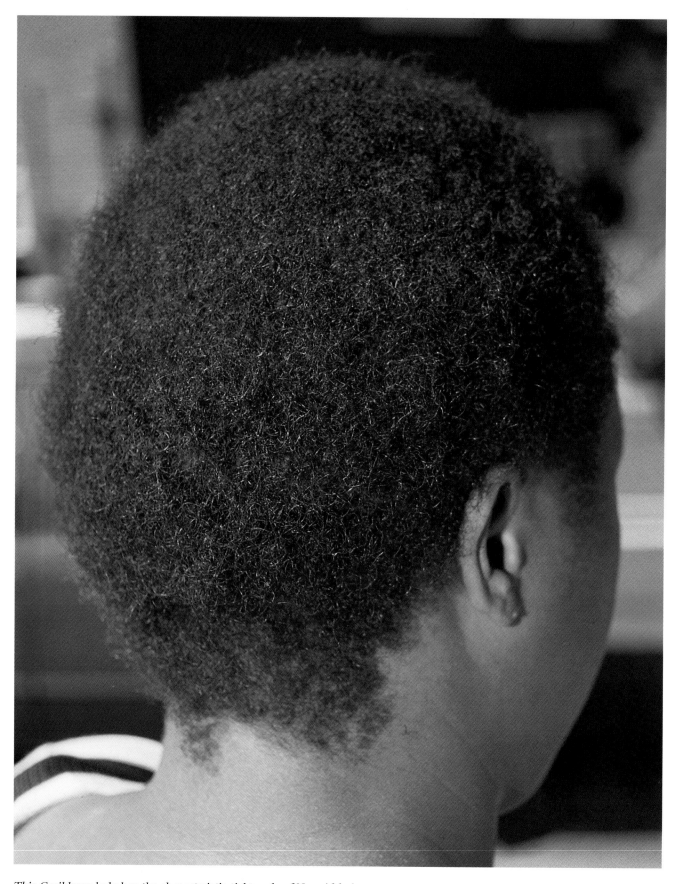

This Caribbean lady has the characteristic tight curls of Negroid hair

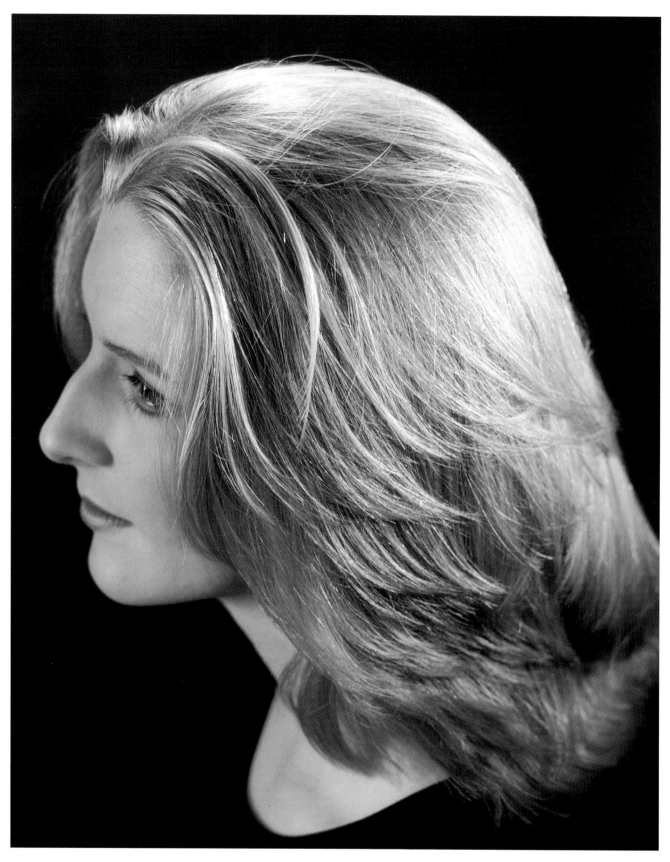

Archetypal Caucasoid hair, never tinted or permed: light is reflected off the intact cuticles to give an appearance of truly 'healthy hair'

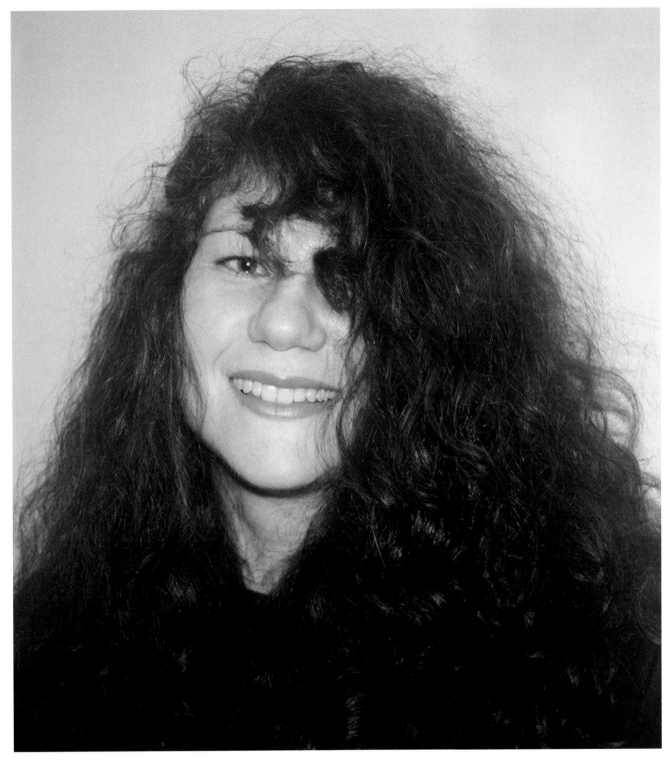

Dark, wavy and plentiful Caucasoid hair – this lady can trace her ancestry to true Gypsies who originated in India and spread through Europe over many hundreds of years

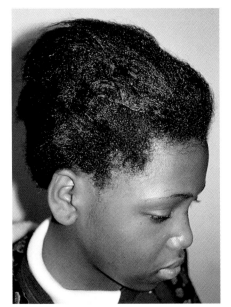

Negroid hair, relaxed and oiled

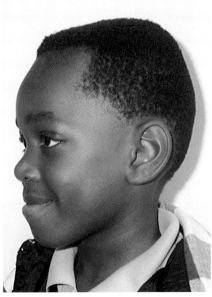

The characteristic tight woolly curls of Negroid hair

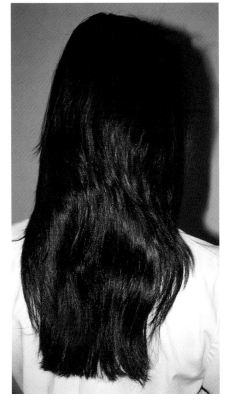

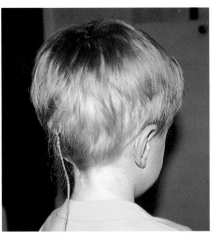

Young Caucasoid hair, showing terminal hairs capable of long anagen

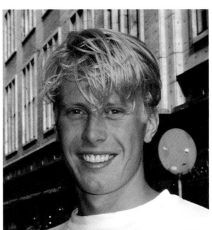

Caucasoid hair can be bleached by the sun

Flowing dark Caucasoid hair, common in people from the Indian subcontinent

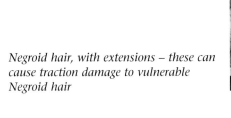

Negroid hair, with extensions – these can cause traction damage to vulnerable Negroid hair

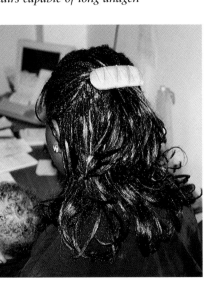

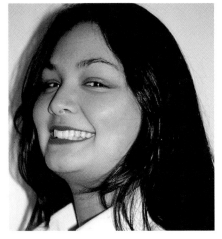

Mixed Mongolian and Caucasoid hair

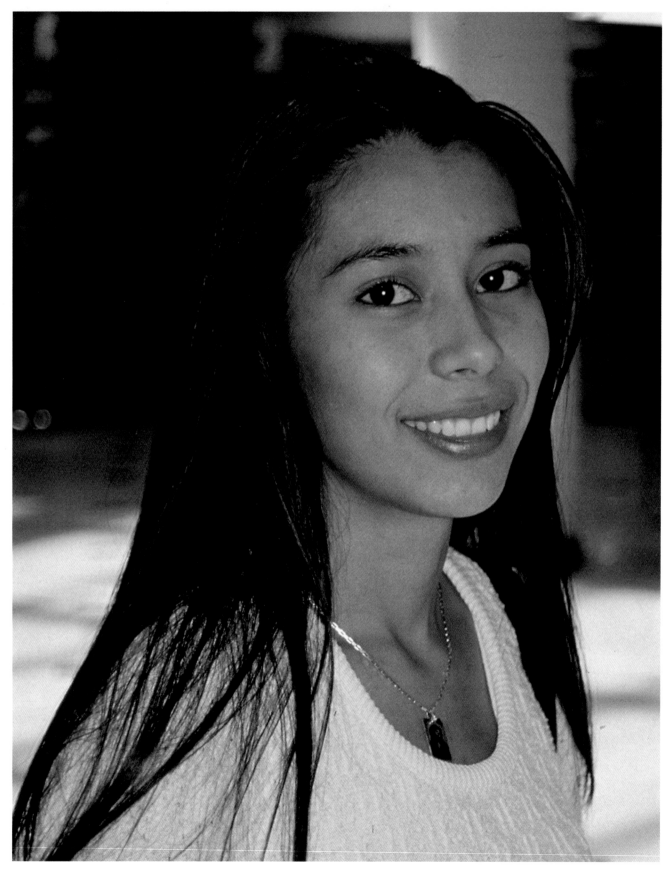

Another Mongoloid/Caucasoid combination – the perfect mixture to produce beautiful hair

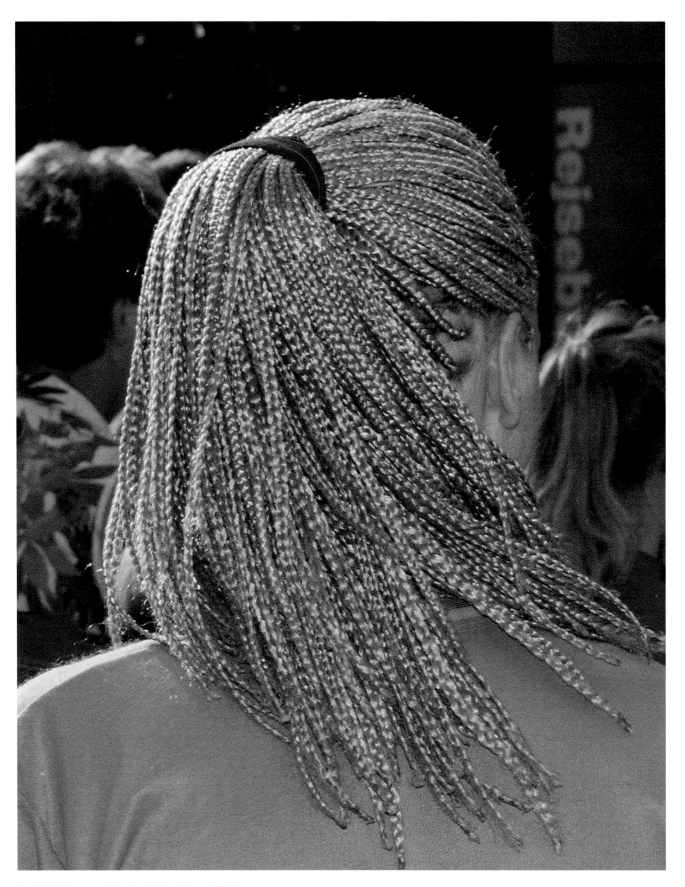

Braided Caucasoid hair mimics Negroid hair

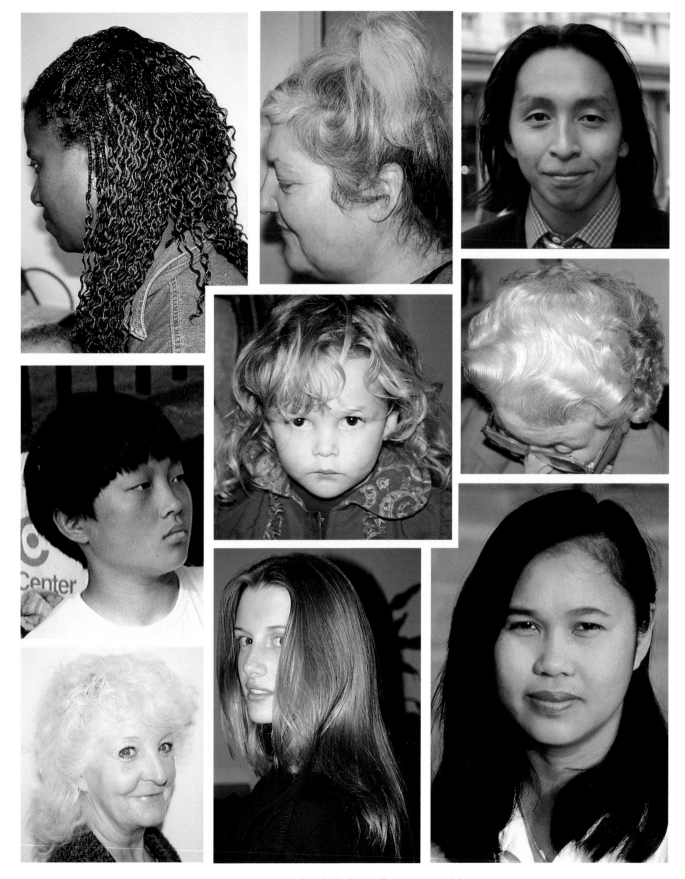

Hair types (and styles!) from all over the world

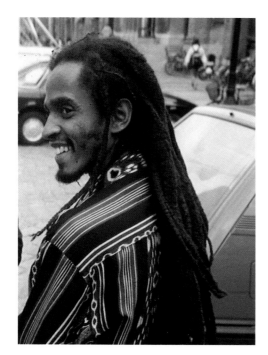

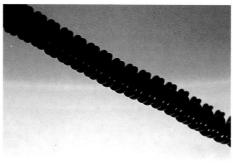

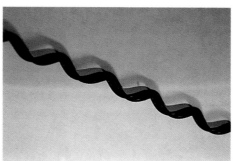

The tight crimped curls of Negroid hair derive from its twisted structure, like that of a spring (above); relaxing (see page 92) slackens the springy structure, reducing the number of twists per centimetre

Variations in structure

Scientists do not fully understand why the different types of hair grow straight or curly or wavy. This is probably determined by several factors, which may vary in their importance during life. This is why some curly-headed children have straight hair later in life, and vice versa. These factors include:

- the way the large bundles of keratin are arranged within each hair shaft
- the position of the hair bulb in the hair follicle – in Negroid hair the bulb may lie to the side of the follicle, and so the hair shaft grows out of the follicle at an acute angle
- irregular growth in the hair bulb – if it varies slightly to one side or the other the hair may grow wavy
- the shape of the hair follicle, whether it is straight or curved
- the number of twists per unit length.

All hair, even the apparently perfectly straight hair of Mongoloid people, twists as it grows. The number of twists in a given length of hair determine how curly it is: the more twists there are, the curlier it will be. Some Negroid hair has 12 times as many twists per centimetre as Caucasian hair.

In Mongoloid people the keratin bundles in the hair are all straight. The hair shaft tends to be thick, and almost completely round.

The keratin bundles in the hair of Caucasoid people are a mixture: most are straight, some are wavy. The proportions of the two types vary a lot. The hair shaft is usually oval in shape.

The tightly curled hair of Negroid people twists much more frequently than in the other groups. The hair shafts are markedly oval in shape, with definite edges. The cuticle is sharply kinked at the edges, and is especially easily damaged at these points. This curious shape is the reason for the vulnerability of Negroid hair to all forms of physical and chemical trauma, and its consequent need for extreme care in handling and very thorough conditioning.

Straight hair sometimes becomes quite wavy when damp, and wavy hair may become

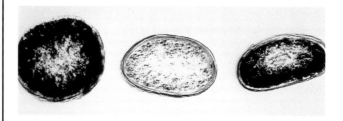

Compare these cross-sections of three hairs, all of different racial types: (left) Mongoloid, (centre) Caucasoid, (right) Negroid

straight when thoroughly doused with water – in a swimming pool, for instance. This is because in these conditions great numbers of hydrogen bonds have been broken. The effect is very temporary, and the hair recovers on drying.

Mixed types
Over many thousands of years these three groups of people have intermingled. Their descendants now show every imaginable blend of hair type and colour, as illustrated on pages 43–4, 51 and 53.

Straight or curly?
Of the three racial groups, the Caucasoids are by far the most varied in the appearance of their hair. It may fall completely straight, it may be crinkly or wavy, or it may form large curls, or pretty well anything in between. Blondes tend to have straight hair, while more brunettes have curly hair. The longer the hair grows, the more obvious its basic character becomes. The first month or two's growth of a new hair may be straight, but then it may start to curl or wave.

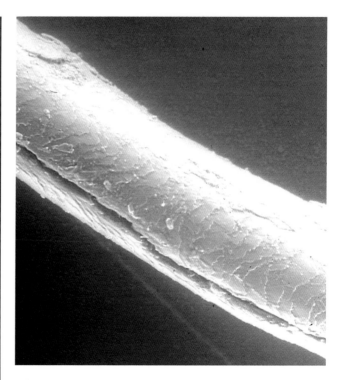

African hair (electronmicrograph): the longitudinal grooving is very common in this type of hair

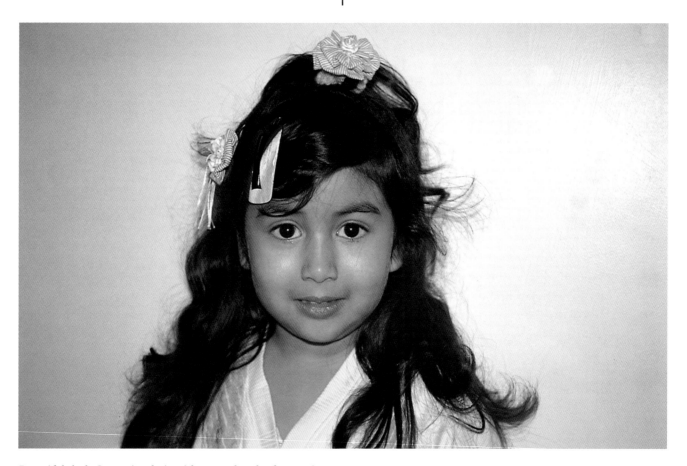

Beautiful dark Caucasian hair with natural curls, from India

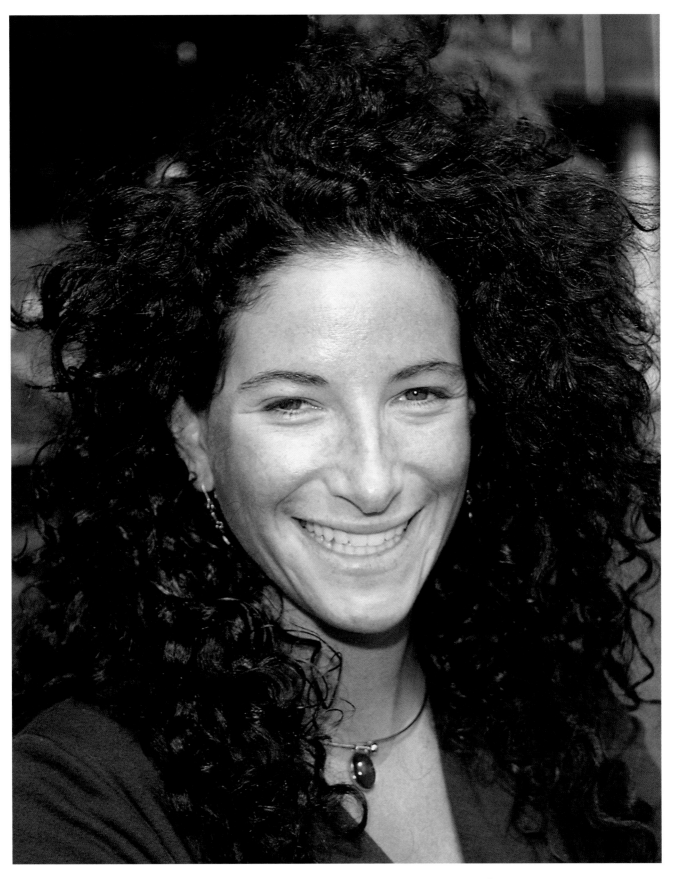

A stunning mass of natural curls: this lady's great-grandparents came from eastern Europe and Russia

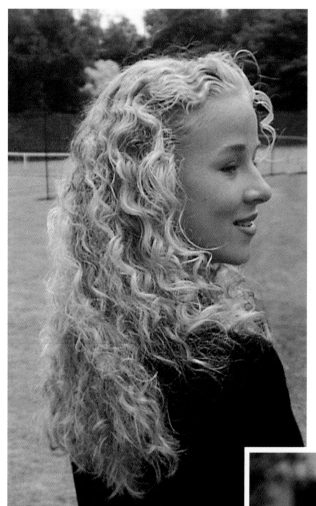

Masses of naturally curly Caucasoid hair…

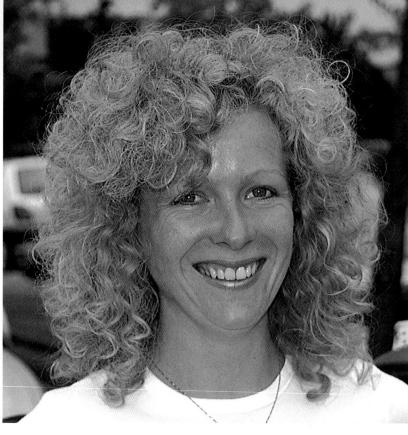

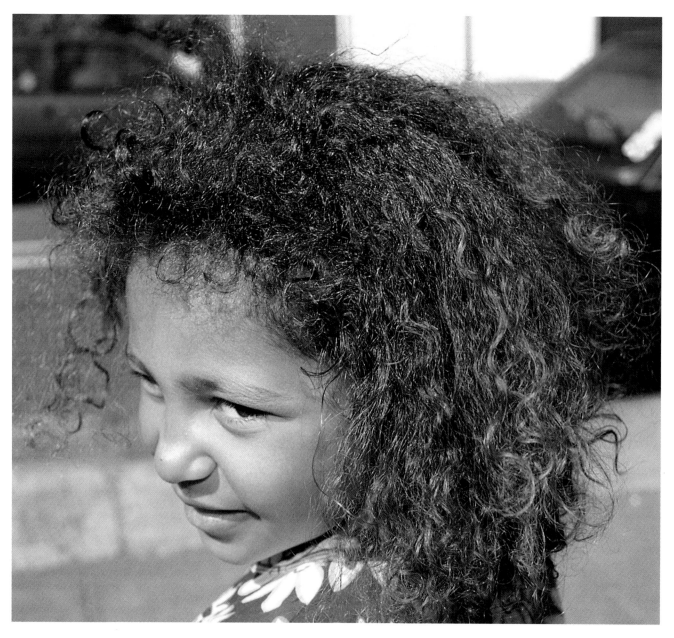

... these curls, however, are of mixed Negroid and Caucasoid types

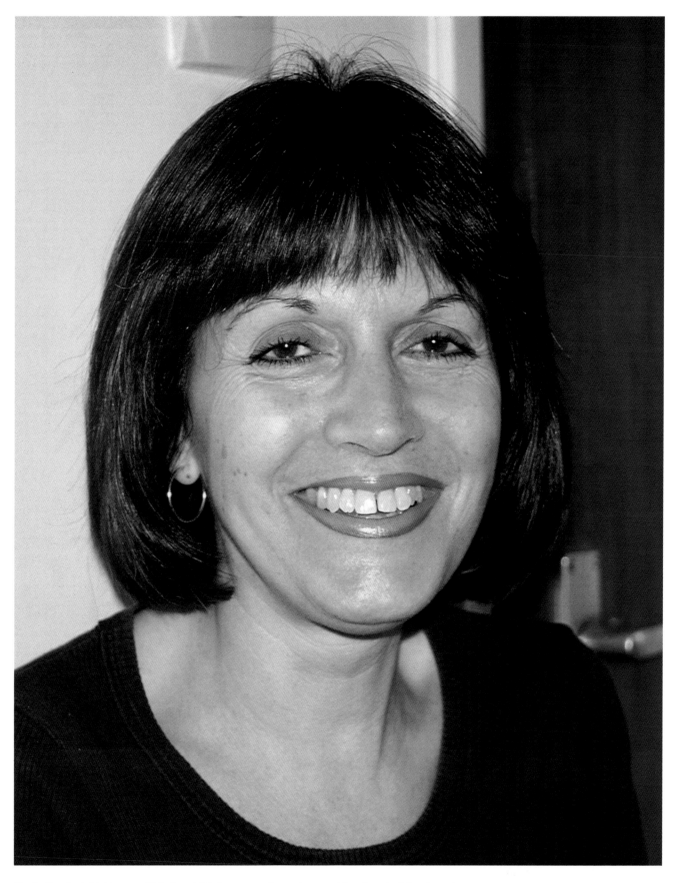

Perfectly straight Caucasoid hair, which has never been damaged by chemical treatment

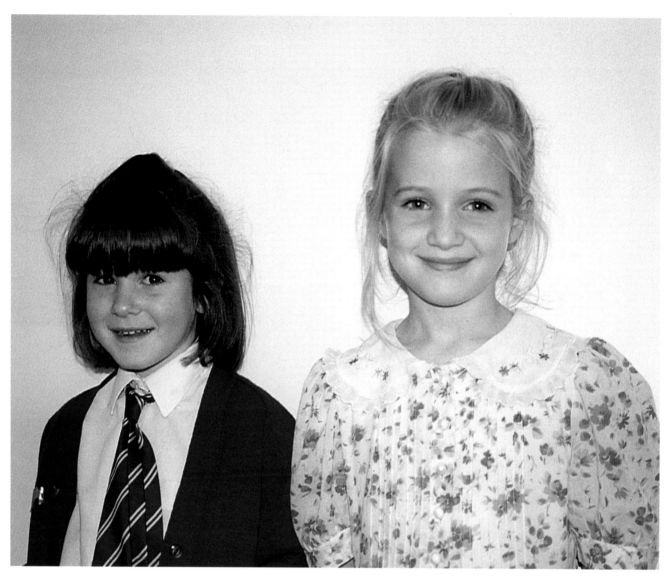

Sisters whose different genetic make-up has led to very different hair types

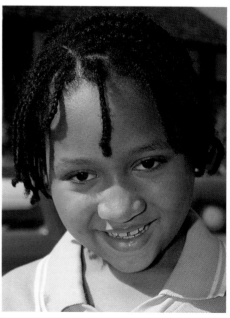

This little girl's hair shows a blending of the Negroid and Caucasoid characteristics she has inherited

Dry or greasy?

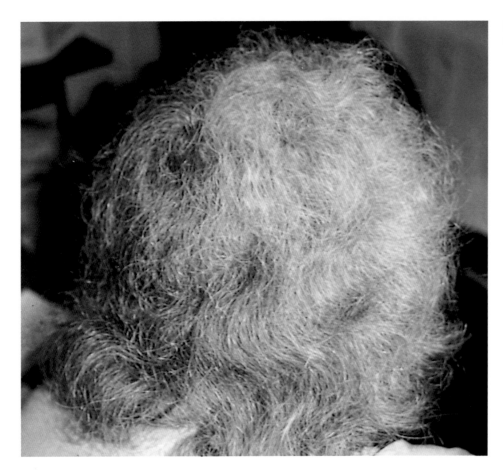

Hair so dry you could probably set fire to it!

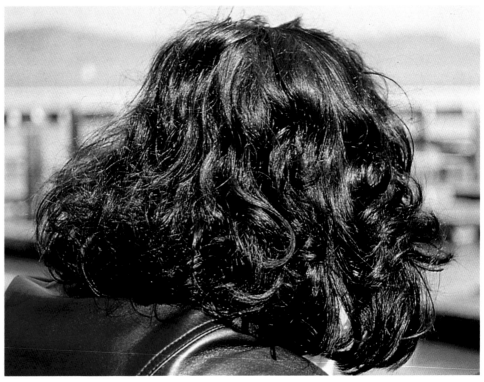

The converse: naturally greasy hair

Dry or greasy?

Greasy hair is due to a build-up of the natural secretion ('grease' or, more correctly, sebum) from glands in the scalp (sebaceous glands). The sebum passes into the hair follicle and spreads upwards and over the hair shaft. It is not absorbed into the shaft.

The feel of the hair depends on the volume of grease present. At certain times, such as puberty, there is a marked change in sebum production due to higher levels of male hormones. At such times the hair may become more greasy and need to be washed more often. Inadequate removal of the grease makes the problem worse.

The scalp produces much the same amount of grease whatever the hair style. Since very short hair offers a smaller area over which the grease can spread, greasiness can be especially troublesome on short hair.

Not shampooing often enough may result in a build-up of grease and material – environmental dirt and bacteria – on the hair. Perspiration plus grease may result in lank strands of hair which look unpleasant and may be unmanageable.

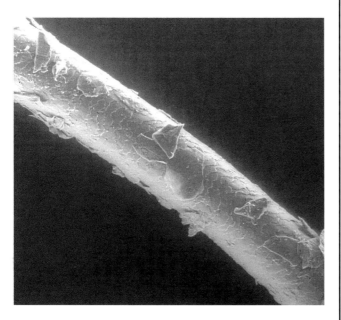

Hair that has not been washed for some time

It is not possible to stop the glands from producing grease. Nor is grease production affected by diet, or indeed by any other factor that we can control. The answer to greasy hair is to wash it as often as necessary to keep it clean and in good condition. Frequent washing does *not* encourage the production of grease. Shampoos designed for greasy hair are specially formulated to remove natural grease without damaging the hair shaft.

Dry hair is hair which does not contain enough moisture. This is usually because the cuticle has become heavily weathered and porous, so that the cortex cannot retain water. It shows up more in long hair than in short, simply because the hair has been growing for longer and therefore has weathered more. It is more common in women than in men, because women are more likely to wear their hair long. The dryness may come to affect more of the hair if it is given repeated chemical treatments, particularly perming, and especially perming associated with bleaching.

Dry hair *feels* dry. It does not shine and is difficult to style. It responds to intensive conditioning, however. Conditioners (see page 132) protect the edges of the cuticle scales, although they cannot cure split ends where the cortex has burst out. Careful brushing, drying and combing after washing are important.

Modern hair products designed for dry hair have large molecules containing positive electrical charges. Hairs carry a small negative charge, so the charged molecules cling to the hairs. They collect on the edges of the damaged scales of the cuticle, helping to smooth over and fill in the breaks and cracks. As a result the hair tends to become more manageable and shiny. Proteins and dimethicone are useful in this process.

In addition panthenol, derived from vitamin B, is absorbed into the shaft and provides moisture. It also penetrates the scalp and reaches the hair follicle itself, improving the moisture content of the hair as soon as it starts to grow.

A Malaysian lady, unusual in having naturally greasy hair

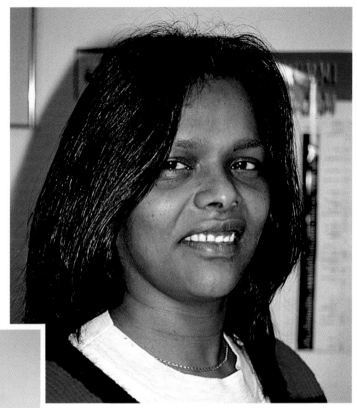

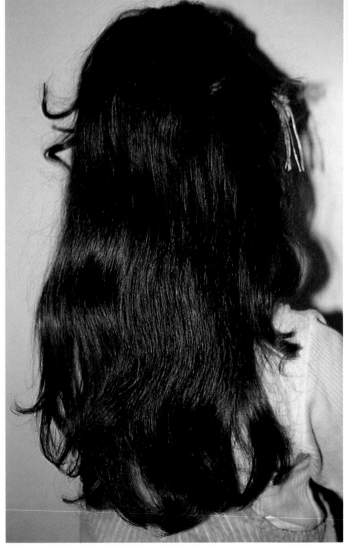

In this young girl, sebum production is not yet influenced by androgens

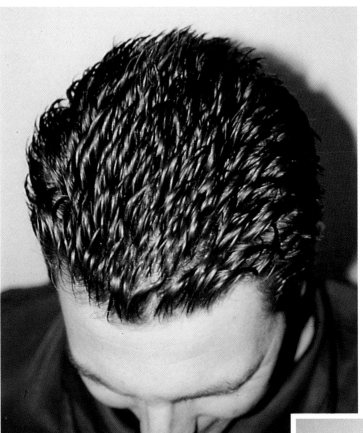

Some people like to add oils to their hair, with the aim of producing extra gloss and shine

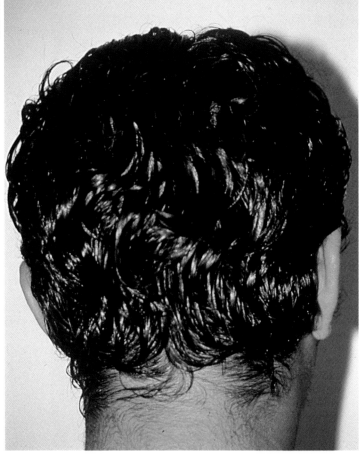

Hair colour

Masses of pigment!...

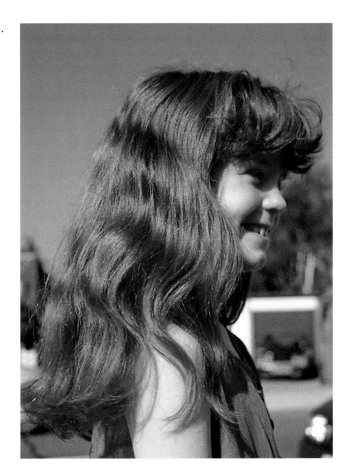

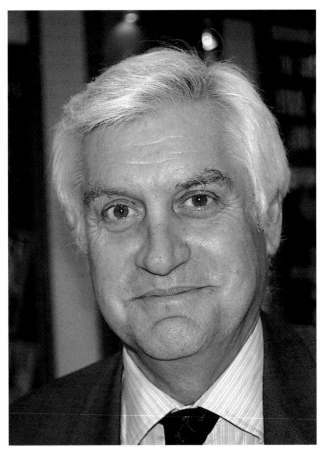

... but here pigment production has virtually ceased, resulting in a distinguished head of silver hair

Hair colour

Pigmentation

Colour is perhaps the most obvious characteristic of hair, but as far as we know it has no biological function in humans. It does not protect the hair from the harmful effects of sunlight (although hair itself protects the scalp, of course).

As we have seen, the colour of hair is due to the presence in the cortex of granules of a pigment called melanin, which is formed in special pigment-producing cells (melanocytes) in the hair bulb during the growing phase (anagen) of each hair. The melanin granules lie along the amino acid chains of the proteins, looking under the microscope rather like a string of pearls.

Melanin is found in two forms. **Eumelanin** is the dark pigment which predominates in black and brunette hair. **Phaeomelanin** is a lighter pigment, which is found in red and blond hair. Many people's hair contains a mixture of the two: the more eumelanin there is in the mixture, the darker is the hair. The mixture (and the shade) varies not only from one person to another, but also across one person's head. The combination of pigments in the mixture is determined by the individual's genes. Differences between dark-haired people are due to differences in the overall quantities of melanins in their hair.

Eumelanin granules are oval (elliptical) in shape, fairly uniform in their make-up and quite hard, with sharply defined edges. Phaeomelanin granules are smaller, partly oval and partly rod-shaped.

The range of colours produced by melanins is limited to shades of yellow, brown, red and black. Grey hairs contain only a few melanin granules, spread out through the hair. White hairs contain no melanin at all: their whiteness is an optical effect, due to the way they reflect the light. Surprisingly, however, unpigmented hairs look yellow (the 'colour' of keratin) when they first grow, and only later turn white.

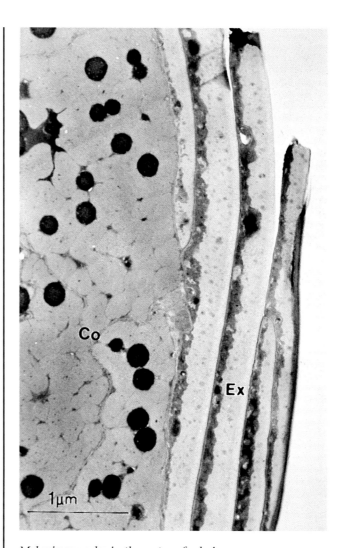

Melanin granules in the cortex of a hair

Genetic differences

Ethnic differences in hair colour are as obvious as are differences in hair type. Most people in the world have dark hair, though in northern Europe blond hair is the most common. Curiously, however, people with blond hair and/or blue eyes are found even in North Africa and the Middle East.

Melanin distribution

Melanin granules are spread out throughout the cortex of the hair. There are more of them near the outer edge of the cortex than towards the middle. The darker the hair, the more melanin granules it contains.

Effects of weathering

The ends of the hair may look lighter than the rest, because of the normal weathering that affects everyone's hair. Heavily weathered hair, which is often brittle, tends to look lighter too.

Red hair

Red hair is relatively uncommon in Europe, except in Scotland: more than one in ten Scots are redheads. Red-haired people often have pale skin that burns easily.

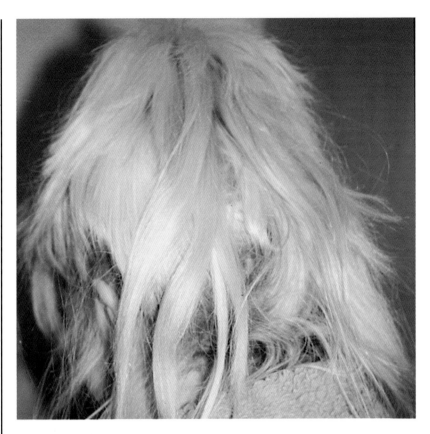

Seriously weathered hair: she needs to see a stylist, urgently!

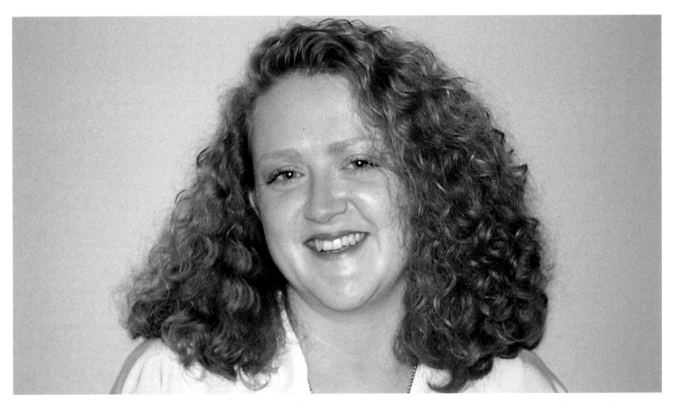

This woman's coloration is typically Celtic: her hair pigment consists overwhelmingly of phaeomelanin, her skin is freckled and tends to burn easily, and her eyes are blue

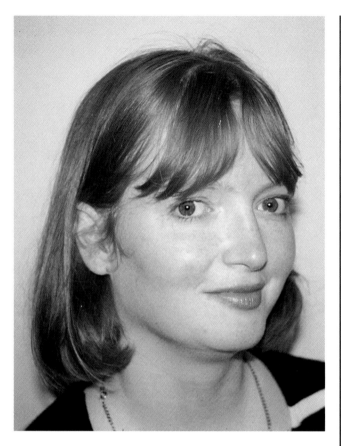

One in ten Scots have red hair

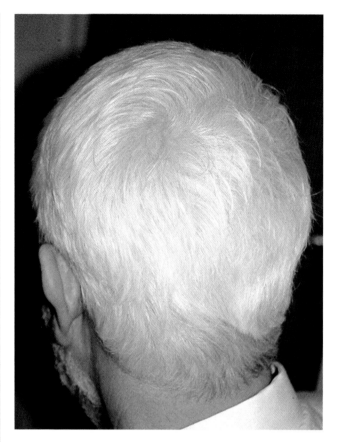

Hair with no pigment at all

In red hair, nearly all the melanin is present in the form of phaeomelanin. Colouring red hair is difficult because of this different pigmentation, and bleaching red hair to a lighter shade is especially hard.

Greying hair

Grey hair is one of the most familiar signs of ageing. The age when greying starts depends on one's genetic inheritance. But in half of all Caucasoid people, half the hairs on the scalp are grey by the age of 50.

The loss of hair colour is due to a gradual fall in melanin production in the hair bulb. If you look at the hairs on a greying head you find a full range of colour, from the normal shade through to white along each hair, and also from one hair to another. Usually people notice their first grey hairs near their temples. Then the greyness spreads to the crown, and later to the back of the head.

Rapid greying

You have probably heard stories about people who are supposed to have 'gone white overnight' following some terrible shock or grief. Treat these tales with caution! A black hair cannot of itself suddenly turn white. Hairs grow for years with pigment inside them, and since they are 'dead' there is no process by which the melanin throughout a hair can be naturally destroyed rapidly (although it may be bleached by sunlight over many years).

Apparent rapid greying may be due to a selective shedding of pigmented hair in a person who has some grey hairs which are retained. Shedding of this kind usually takes several months, but can happen within a few days. If it does take place quickly the effects can be dramatic, since the person's grey hairs may not have been at all obvious until the darker hairs were lost.

Whether stress or shock can cause this kind of hair loss (known as **alopecia areata**) is unknown.

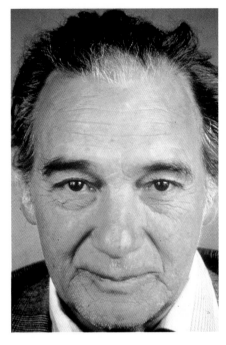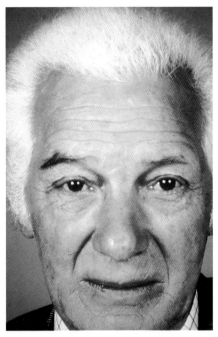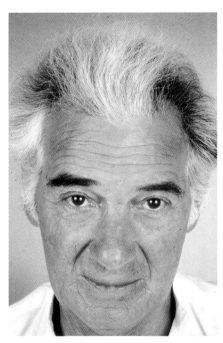

This gentleman's hair went grey very quickly, almost in the legendary 'overnight' fashion. (Left) His hair was naturally a mixture of pigmented and unpigmented (white) hairs, the so-called 'salt and pepper' look. (Centre) In an acute episode of alopecia areata he lost the pigmented hairs, leaving only the unpigmented ones. (Right) He recovered spontaneously, and when his hair re-grew the 'salt and pepper' mixture returned

Premature greying

Very rarely, an individual's hair may begin to turn grey at an unexpectedly early age – before the age of 20 in Caucasoids and before 30 in Negroids. In some people the cause is a medical condition. More usually it is due to the presence of a particular gene.

Albinism

Albinism is an inherited condition in which there is little or no pigment in the hair. An albino's hair is startlingly pale, either light yellow or nearly white. Albino skin is also pale, even in Negroid people.

Where the condition is severe the eyes lack pigment too, and look pink: albino people often have poor vision.

Acquired colour defects

Inflammation in the hair follicle, which can occur in shingles, damages the melanocytes and may lead to loss of hair colour. So too may exposure to X-rays, though very rarely a deeper colour develops. Occasionally white patches form in the beard after dental treatment.

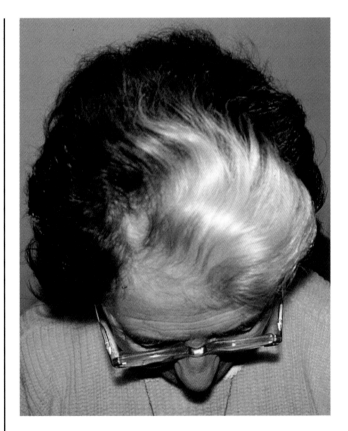

This lady developed the silver streak in her hair before she was twenty – as did her mother: the feature is genetically determined

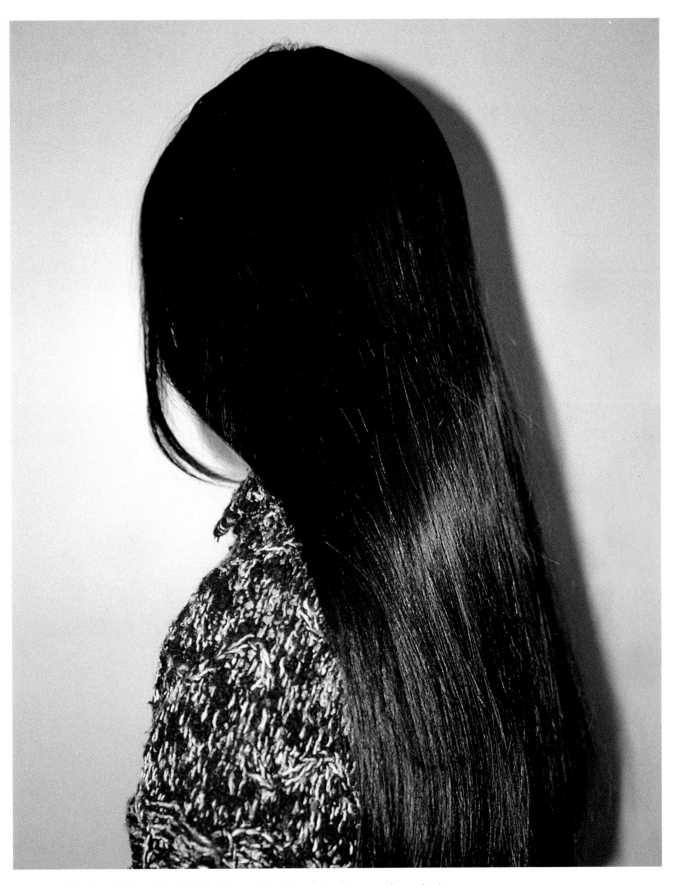

The beautiful black hair of this Asian lady owes its colour to high levels of eumelanin

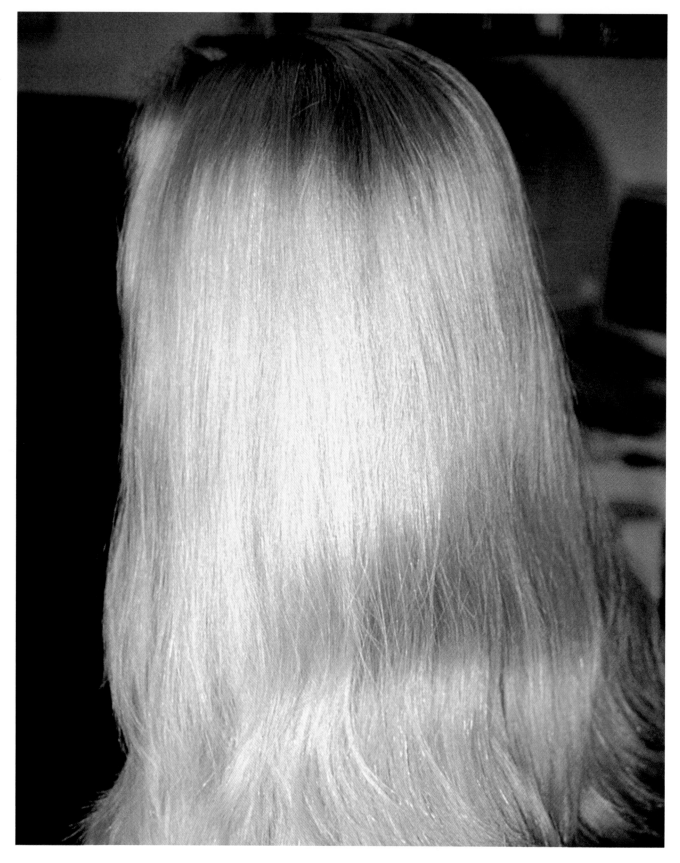

Fabulous healthy hair! The way it reflects light indicates intact hair cuticles, and speaks of the routine use of good-quality hair products

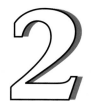

Hair care

About this chapter ...

In this chapter we deal with the basic scientific principles behind keeping hair 'in good condition'. We look at what is meant by 'good condition', and why hair sometimes gets into 'bad condition'.

We present some 'dos and don'ts', and look at a few real-life examples.

Hair condition

Hair is a remarkably tough material. It can stand up to considerable abuse, but over time this can wreak havoc with its natural properties. In particular, its porosity can be badly affected, so that it breaks easily and cannot be styled satisfactorily.

On the other hand, we can recognise hair that is in good condition. It shines, it is easy to manage – it just looks good. Even though the hair shaft is technically 'dead', in that its cells are no longer dividing, we may describe it as 'healthy'. So why can its properties change so much that the hair loses this 'healthy' appearance?

Sometimes this may be due to a medical condition such as poor nutrition: starvation or anaemia due to a lack of protein in the diet can damage the hair. In famine conditions, some people's hair changes as it grows from black to gingery-red if they cannot get enough protein.

We have seen that in older people hair may not be able to grow as long as it used to, and may become thinner and lose its pigmentation. It might be thought to be less healthy. But it can still maintain its structure, and indeed many elderly people have beautiful hair.

Probably the most obvious aspect of healthy hair is its shine – its ability to reflect light. This property depends mainly on the cuticle of the hair shaft, and how intact it is.

So the good condition of your hair in fact depends on the current state of each of the 100,000 or so individual hair shafts on your head. If the cuticles are intact, if their cortex has not been affected by heat or chemicals, and if

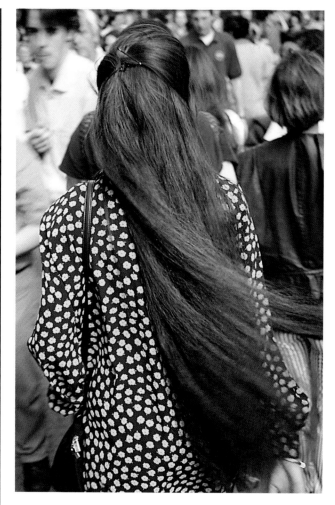

Hair this long must have been growing for seven or eight years: just look at its beautiful condition

the hair is not caked with grease and old hair spray, then the hair will probably have reasonable shine and body.

Hair in good condition

In the end, the condition of hair depends on what is done to it. You are your own hair's worst enemy!

By the time your hair reaches your shoulders, it has probably been growing for three years or more. Hair that is level with your waist is around five years old (at least at the tip). If you are lucky enough to have hair long enough to sit on, that hair may be as much as a dozen years old. And throughout its growth it needs to be cared for to keep its healthy look. A damaged cuticle cannot heal, because the scales are 'dead', although much can be done to help its appearance.

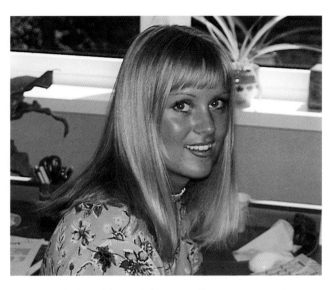

The straight blond hair of this tanned young woman is naturally sun-bleached, and reflects light well

If you are sensible, you clean your hair frequently, using good-quality products, and – most importantly – remember to **condition** it well. You have the ends cut regularly by a skilled stylist, so as to prevent weathering effects such as split ends. If you are thinking of changing its colour you get advice first from an experienced hair technician, who can tell you how much colour change your particular hair can stand, and which products would be suitable. If you are considering a perm you ask for advice on whether your hair type can stand perming at the moment, or if it would be safer to improve its condition first. And, once permed, you pay even more attention to conditioning your hair, and you don't repeat the perm too often.

With an understanding of the principles of good hair care, and regularly putting those principles into practice, everyone can aim to keep their hair in good condition.

Hair in poor condition

The natural look of your hair depends on several inherited factors. Hair that is in poor condition looks dull and dry. So how does it get that way?

Dark hair, as we have seen, looks glossier than blond hair. The presence or absence of natural oils makes a difference. And very straight hair reflects light better than tousled hair does.

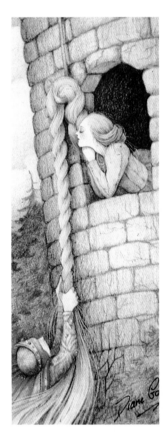

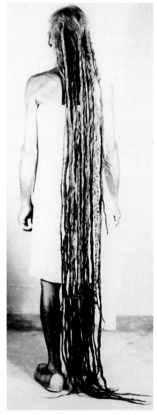

The golden hair of the imprisoned fairy-tale princess Rapunzel was long enough to allow her lover to climb it in order to reach her in her tower – a demonstration not only of the length of anagen in Rapunzel, but also of the inherent strength of hair

This man is head of a religious cult which requires its leader to be able to grow his hair long enough to reach the ground: his anagen period is probably around ten or twelve years. As he grows older and the anagen period shortens, he may lose his job

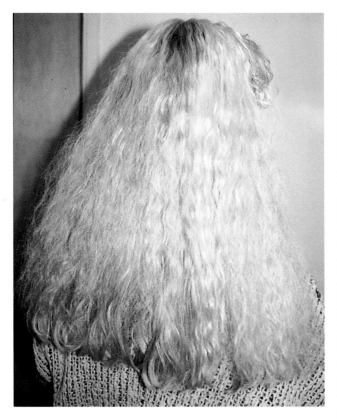

Long hair that has been bleached and permed needs the most conditioning

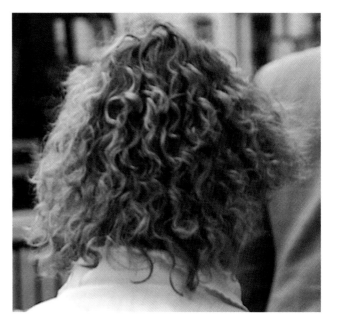

Very neglected, processed hair: a conditioner is essential!

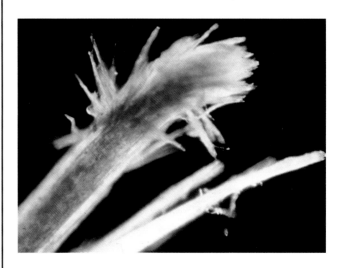

A classical split end, with gross disruption of the cortex

Some of us, however, fall into the trap of trying to improve upon nature, not just once but over and over again. Where you can go wrong includes:

- not understanding the basic properties of hair in general, and your own hair in particular
- trying to lighten the colour of your hair more than it can stand (bleach damage)
- continually trying to correct previous mistakes
- perming hair that is already in poor condition.

Hair damage

In this section we look at some real-life cases of hair that is obviously not in good condition.

This person's hair looks dull and lifeless. It doesn't shine, and it is obviously difficult to manage. Examining a few hairs under the microscope would reveal what has happened to it, and suggest what might be done.

It is all too easy to fall into the trap of blaming the last product put on to the hair as the single cause of a problem. Much more often, hair condition is lost as a result of a combination of mis-treatments over a long period.

Damage from weathering

Weathering, as you saw in Chapter 1, is the gradual wearing away of the cuticle of the hair shaft. The damage exposes the cortex, which becomes worn down as well, and the hair can eventually break. Fortunately, hair is tough by nature: hairs taken from ancient Egyptian mummies and even from the bodies of our Stone Age ancestors look remarkably well preserved after thousands of years. Many of us have hair that withstands reasonably well most of the abuse we seem determined to throw at it.

But in spite of this resilience, badly weathered hair is quite common. All too often it results in disappointment and an unhappy client for the stylist and the technician to sort out. But whatever their expertise, repeated attempts to restore the hair to good condition by further experiment may be doomed to failure. All hair has its limit: once that limit is passed and the hair has seriously broken down, the only thing to be done is to cut it off.

When new hair first grows up out of the scalp, the cuticle consists of up to ten layers of long 'scales'. Even so, it is incredibly thin – only 3 or 4 μm – and it has to last for maybe six years or more. As the hair grows, the layers are little by little worn down. At the end of the

hair, especially if it is long, they have worn almost completely away.

This wearing is a perfectly natural process, and has little effect on the hair. But it is very much speeded up by some of the things that happen to the hair. These can include wetting, friction, sunlight, heat from hair dryers or the sun, chemicals in swimming pools and salt in seawater, as well as cosmetic procedures of various kinds, are just some of these.

The photograph below shows what a new hair looks like under the electron microscope. It shows the regular layers of cuticle scales overlying the cortex in long, smooth curves.

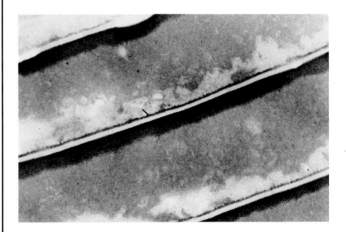

The next photograph shows (on a much smaller scale) an area further down the same hair. Here the scales have started to become chipped and broken in places. This is quite normal: it results from ordinary combing, which rubs the hair down its length, producing friction as it goes. The gentle friction of hairs rubbing against each other also produces some damage.

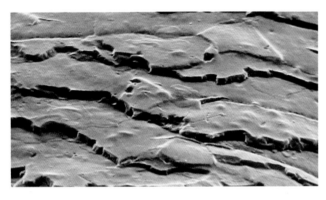

Very highly magnified electronmicrograph of normal cuticles, showing how the scales overlap (the scale run from the base of the hair towards the tip)

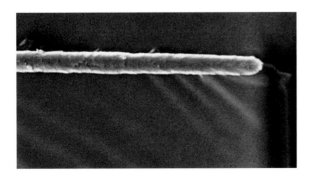

The tip of a normal hair that has been normally weathered

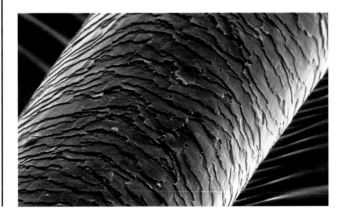

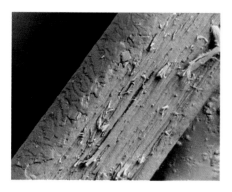

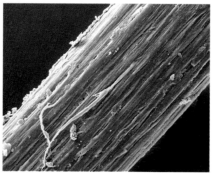

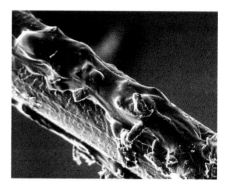

The continuing destruction of the cortex of a hair: the long parallel bundles of keratin have been exposed and can be seen clearly

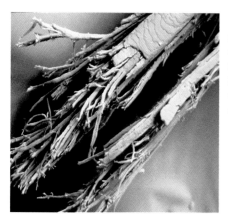

The cortex has ruptured and cannot be repaired, so that the only course of action is to cut off the hair

The use of good-quality scissors is a vital part of hair care

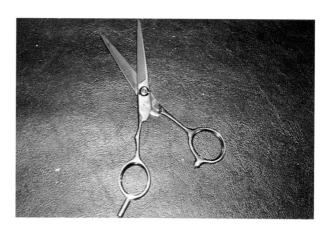

In the photographs above some more serious harm can be seen. Large areas of the cuticle have split away, showing the cortex underneath. This is how the classic 'split end' starts, with a crack beginning to run back up the hair shaft.

If the problem is really severe, the cortex bursts right out of the hair.

In normal hair, this sort of damage is only noticeable near the tips of untrimmed long hair, which may look lustreless and pale with some split ends. The length of time for which hair can grow without the damage becoming visible depends on the natural quality of the hair, how frequently it is damaged, and how much on-going protection has been given to it by conditioning.

The reason why conditioning is so important in slowing down natural weathering lies in the ability of the cortex to retain moisture. Dry, out-of-condition hair lacks moisture, and the correct moisture content (**hydration**) of hair has to be restored for the hair to regain its condition and its 'healthy' look. Without enough moisture the number of hydrogen bonds may be reduced.

Conditioning allows re-establishment of the hydrogen bonds and improves the moisture content of the hair by improving the weatherproofing of the cuticle. This determines the amount of static charge on the hair and the resistance of hair to mechanical stresses like brushing and combing.

Damage from hair cutting and styling

Cutting hair with blunt scissors results in a cut with a long, jagged edge, at which the cuticle scales will be especially vulnerable to further damage. This is why stylists use good-quality steel scissors, which are very sharp indeed and cut cleanly. It is even possible to tell whether a stylist chose to use scissors or a razor by looking at the record of the hair: razor cutting produces long, tapering sections of cuticle which weather quickly, and even peel back.

Some stylists prefer to cut hair when it is dry, in the belief that this will save the hair from heavy brushing when it is damp and therefore vulnerable to damage. A circular or semicircular brush is probably the least damaging to hair.

HAIR FACTS

Hair carries its history

The hair shaft carries a unique historical record of everything that has happened to it during its long growth. As a hair grows, the year-on-year accumulation of the effects of drying, dyeing, colouring and so forth are recorded in its structure, and the record can be 'read 'under the microscope.

One way of looking at how long this record stays on the hair is to measure the length of the hair (assuming that it grows by a centimetre a month) and marking past world events along its length.

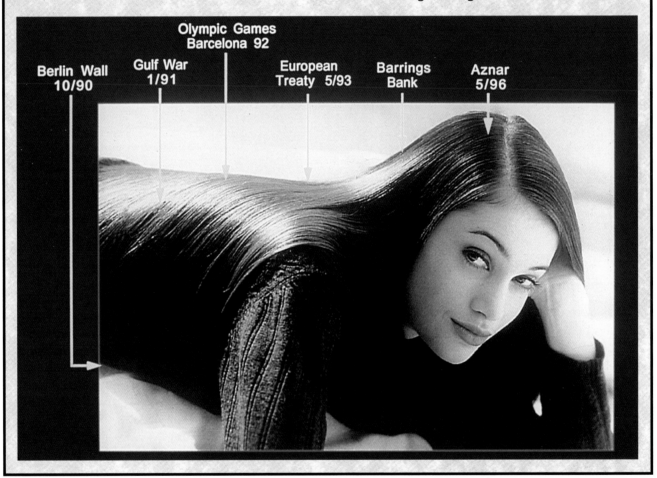

Berlin Wall 10/90 • Gulf War 1/91 • Olympic Games Barcelona 92 • European Treaty 5/93 • Barrings Bank • Aznar 5/96

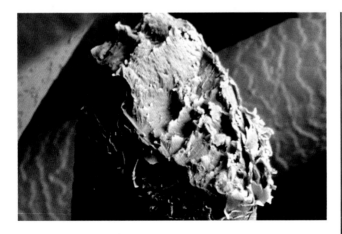

The stump of a hair that has been badly cut

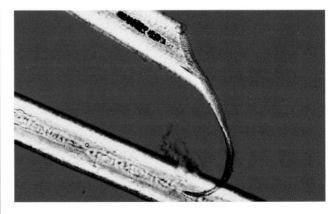

Unskilled razor cutting can leave a long 'tail' on the severed hair, which may lead to breakdown of the end of the hair

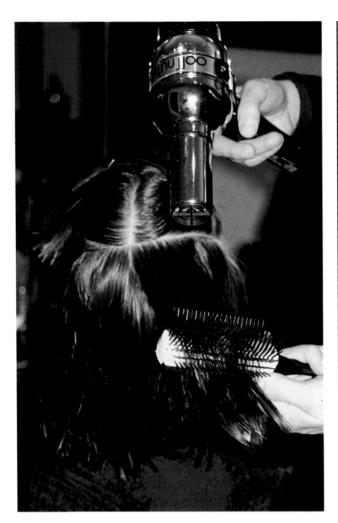

Careful blow drying on a moderate setting should not damage the hair – but if this dryer is set on maximum heat it may be too close to the hair

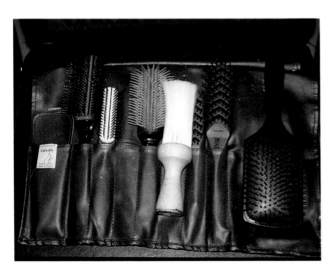

Some of the tools of the hairdresser's trade – notice the broad brushes, which are 'kind' to the hair

Damage from hair treatments

Shampooing should not in itself damage the hair, since modern shampoos do not lift the cuticle. In the past, when harsh shampoos were often used, acute and irreversible tangling or matting sometimes followed shampooing. The culprits were usually antiseptic shampoos, and they could turn hair into a mass that looked more like sheep's wool than human hair.

This kind of matting is seldom seen nowadays, fortunately, since most modern shampoos contain conditioning agents and help to protect hair. Small amounts of tangling and occasionally matting are still quite common, however, especially in long weathered hair. It generally affects only small locks of hair or even a few adjacent hairs. It may be the result of wetting and drying hair without shampoo, since friction is higher in wet hair than in dry. It can happen when the hair is piled up on top of the head for shampooing – a recipe for tangling if ever there was one.

Of the common cosmetic procedures, permanent waving, bleaching and dyeing all damage the hair to some extent. Permanent

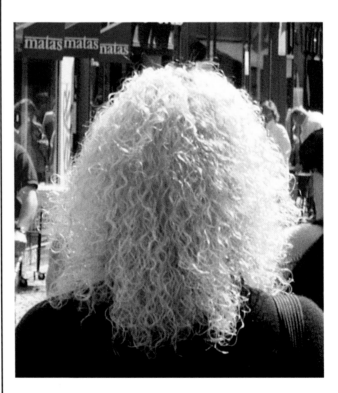

Repeated bleaching and perming will significantly affect the hair's porosity and make it vulnerable to further damage

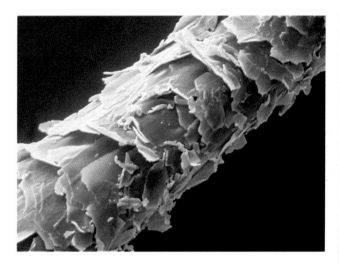

The cuticle of this hair has been significantly damaged by repeated and excessive perming

waving, by its nature, disrupts the structure of the hair: indeed, it has to do so for the perm to be successful. In order to change the shape of the hair, permanent waving agents first break the disulphide bonds that give the hair shaft its structure. The hair is then put into its new shape and 'neutralised'. Neutralisation is the name given to the re-forming of the chemical bonds in their new positions, a process that fixes the hair permanently into its new shape. The secrets of satisfactory perming lie in the manufacturer's formulation of the product and the stylist's expertise in applying the neutralising lotion after just the right length of time, so that the perm is fixed but the hair is damaged as little as possible. Permed hair should always look beautiful in spite of this deliberate 'damage'. (We shall discuss perms in more detail in the next chapter.)

Bleaching and dyeing change hair structure too, because the dyes and the bleaches used have to penetrate the cuticle and get into the cortex where they have their effect. Some degree of chemical damage is unavoidable.

Cosmetic procedures do not damage the hair follicle within the scalp, and so do not cause hair loss. Only a serious chemical burn to the skin of the scalp that destroys the follicle cells can do so. Burns like this can follow indiscriminate over-use of permanent waving or relaxing solutions, and therefore these solutions must be handled carefully at all times.

Damage from the sun

The ultraviolet light in direct sunlight affects the cuticle in a similar way to a bleach, and eventually the keratin protein of the hair breaks down. The result is than the hair is gradually weakened and becomes drier. The effect shows up as light streaks in the hair (sun bleaching). The reason is that sunlight breaks up some of the chemical links within the amino acid groups, in particular those between carbon atoms and sulphur atoms. It does not affect disulphide linkages or hydrogen bonds.

Mechanical damage

Though hair is so robust, it can still be damaged by over-enthusiastic brushing and combing, especially when it is wet and if there is some degree of tangling. Metal combs are particularly hard on the hair. Backbrushing and backcombing are extremely harmful, since they tug against the scales of the cuticle, which all lie pointing towards the tip of the shaft like tiles

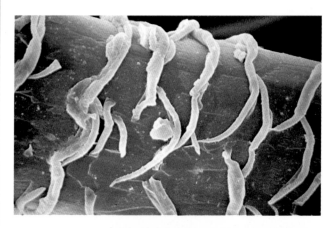

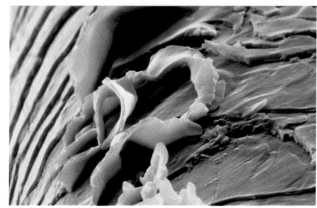

Two views of damage to cuticles, both due to backcombing

on a roof. Once hair has been backcombed the delicate scales are lifted. The next time a comb passes over the scales they will be ripped off. There is no way of repairing this. The effects of these processes can build up over time and cause considerable damage: backcombing is one of the most damaging physical treatments that can be inflicted on hair.

Hair that has been treated chemically (permed, coloured or bleached) has, as we have seen, already been damaged to some extent. The result is that it is at greater risk of damage from the daily hair care routine. The surface of chemically treated hair is receptive to conditioners and other protective treatments, however, and if applied regularly these products can give real protection to the hair.

Heat damage

We have seen the importance of the moisture content of hair to the hair's condition. Processes like blow drying reduce the moisture content below its normal level and can in themselves be harmful. Hair dryers and other heated appliances first soften the keratin of the hair. If they are too hot, they can actually cause the water in the hair to boil, and tiny bubbles of steam then form inside the softened hair shaft. The hair is thereby weakened, and may break altogether. This condition of 'bubble hair' is discussed more fully in Chapter 4.

There is no treatment for seriously heat-damaged hair, although trimming the damaged hair can reduce the formation of split ends.

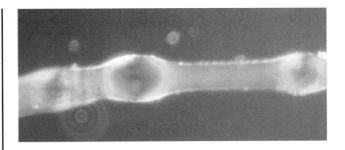

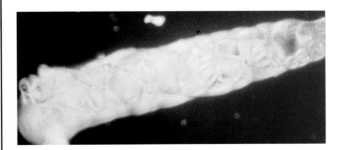

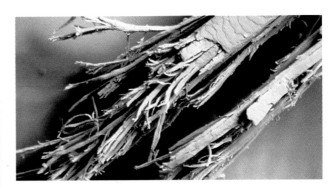

Bubbles formed within hair as a result of water boiling within the cortex

HAIR FACTS

Summary of hair damage

Usually hair damage takes place gradually, stage by stage, as follows:

- the hair is weakened
- the cuticle begins to break down
- the cuticle disappears, layer by layer
- the cortex is exposed
- split ends appear
- the hair breaks.

Minimising damage

Once it has been significantly damaged, the cuticle cannot be repaired. So hair care must be aimed at preventing injury in the first place. Obviously, all procedures should therefore be carried out as gently as possible. Apart from this, the best way to keep damage to a minimum is to condition regularly and thoroughly. This helps to keep the cuticle intact, lower friction and reduce static charge on the hair.

Conditioners that contain **dimethicone** (a silicone compound, made from silica which is one of the commonest substances on earth) deposit mainly at the edges of the cuticle scales – just where the damage happens most easily. Micro-fine droplets make the hair surface

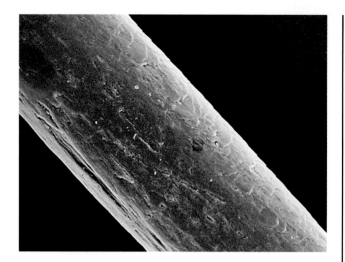

This is Negroid hair (as indicated by the groove along its length): this type of hair, more than any other, needs the protection of conditioning

smooth and shiny (less 'fly-away'). Dimethicone protects the hair from damage by reducing its resistance to brushing, combing and styling, when wet as well as when dry.

Other ingredients in conditioners and other hair care preparations also work to smooth the outer layers of the cuticle. These may include protein extracts (collagen, and the amino acids obtained from silk) and panthenol and similar compounds, which are related to vitamin B5. Some of these are known to penetrate hair and to help to increase its moisture content. Well-conditioned hair is quite easy to de-tangle. Use a large-toothed comb or brush with rounded ends.

The only way to avoid split ends altogether is to use preventive conditioning and to avoid all chemical treatments. Split ends, if they do develop, can never be repaired 'like new'. The so-called 'split end repair fluids' are applied

directly to the hair tips. They contain high-density silicone fluids which draw the splayed ends of the fibres together and hide their ragged appearance. The fluid is removed at the next shampoo, however.

Severe cosmetic damage

Hair that has been badly damaged by cosmetic treatments is surprisingly common. Of course, stylists and technicians are trained to examine hair before carrying out chemical treatment to determine its porosity, and whether there is any possibility of serious damage. But take an enthusiastic amateur embarking on bleaching and perming at home without any basic knowledge or experience, and combine this with a hair dryer used on its hottest setting: you have a recipe for disaster.

Here are a couple of all-too-familiar examples of severe cosmetic damage. Both of them can be avoided by treating the care with the care it deserves.

Trichorrhexis nodosa

This is an explosion of the cortex at a single point on the hair. It looks like a tiny white bead on the hair, and can lead to hair breakage. It is a classic sign of cosmetic and chemical over-treatment of the hair. So its appearance should always prompt the thought, 'What is this person doing to the hair more than the rest of us are doing?

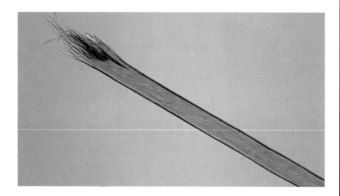

A split end that has been temporarily repaired

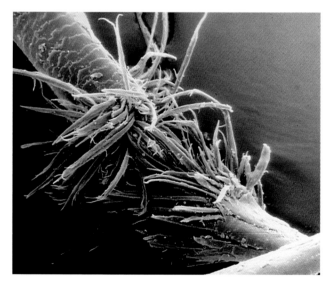

A case of trichorrhexis nodosa, where the cortex was disrupted by an overheated hair dryer

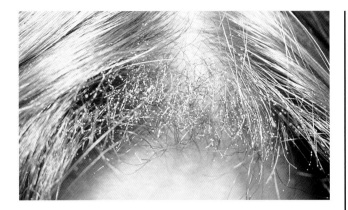

The hair has literally been fried by heat, and then burst open

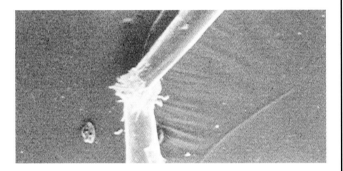

A heat-damaged hair seen under the microscope

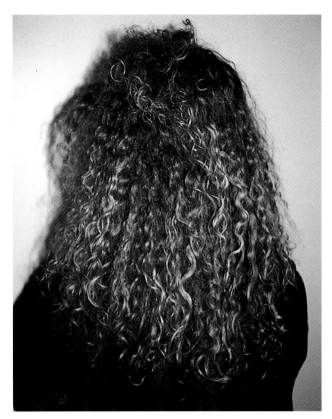

Hair that has been repeatedly permed

Perm damage

A permanent wave process inexpertly applied is probably the most damaging chemical treatment that hairdressers see. This photograph (top right) shows the effect of excessive waving treatment. The cuticle scales on the hair have been lifted up and separated from each other. They will never return to normal, and as soon as a comb passes over them they may break off. The cuticle may be completely stripped off, revealing the cortex underneath. This too is now exposed to weathering, and will probably not survive unbroken for long.

When a new client walks into a salon, the hairdresser never knows what problems are going to face them. A quick assessment reveals whether the client is Caucasian, African, or Asian descent: all these different racial types have different hair qualities and different hair structures. Is this client's hair curly or straight? Dry, greasy or normal? or perhaps of a mixed type? Is it long or short? Thick or thin, in terms of its density on the head? Are the fibres coarse, medium or fine? All these characteristics interact with each other.

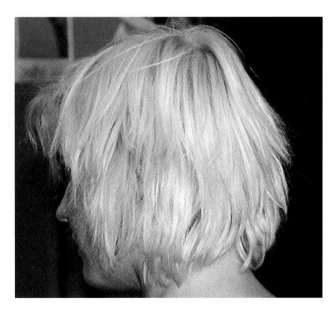

The effects of repeated bleaching, together with unfortunately poor styling

And then, what is the past history of this hair? Has it been permed or bleached, or possibly both?

No two clients are the same. Life in a salon is never dull!

What the eye doesn't see – the good, the bad and the ugly – is made plain by the electron microscope

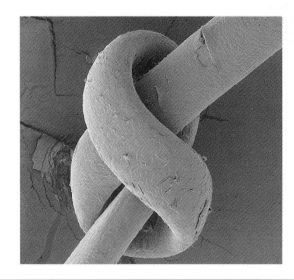

Knotting, associated with Negroid hair…

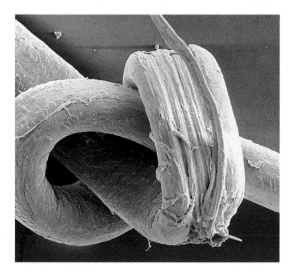

… leads to breakdown

A perfect hair, its cuticle intact, taken from a newborn baby

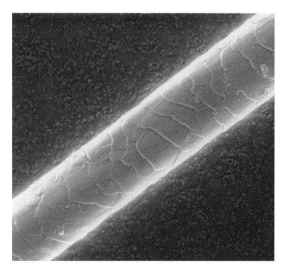

Damaged cuticle, due to backcombing heavily sprayed hair

A hair shattered after severe perm damage

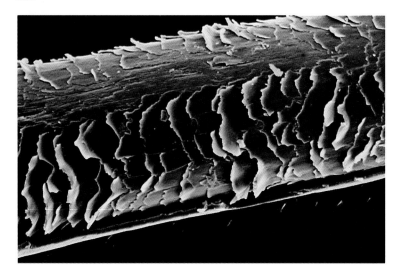

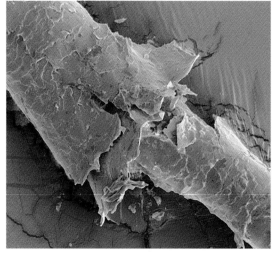

*Hair damage
caused by hair
bands*

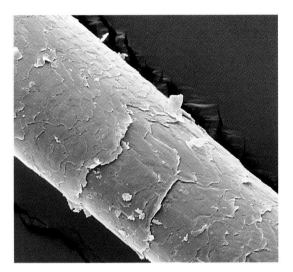

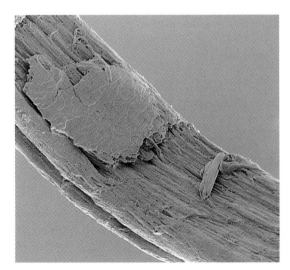

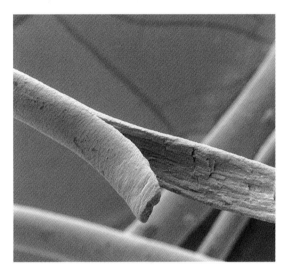

This is the kind of damage that is caused to Negroid hair by the use of chemical relaxants

*In practice, men's hair suffers
less from weathering than
women's hair does, just because
it is usually worn shorter: this is
an exception! Regular styling
and conditioning would help*

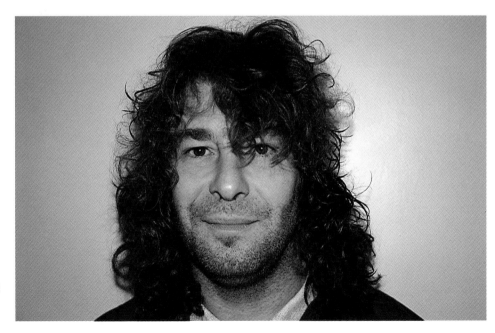

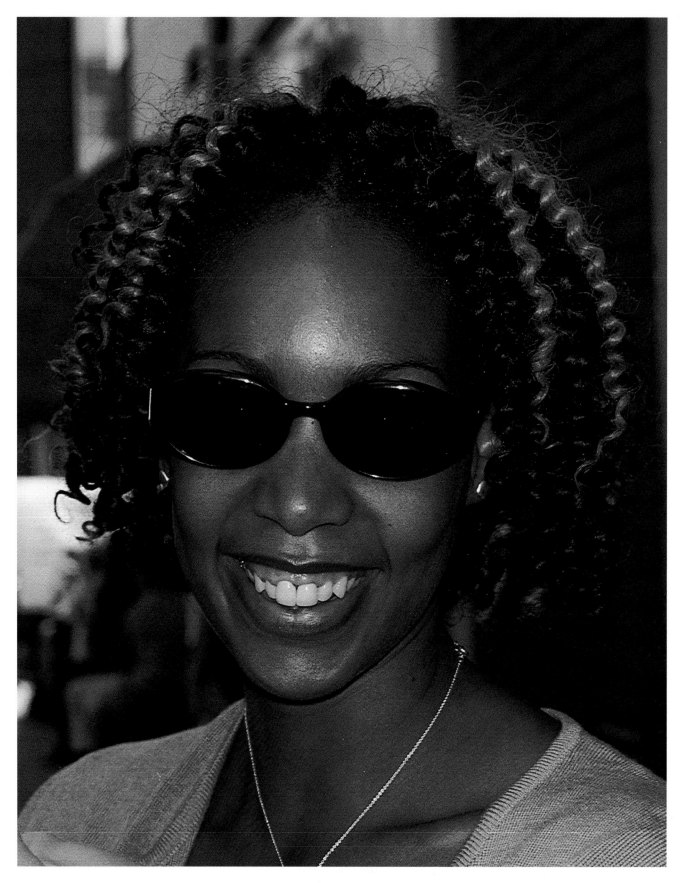

A confident woman who has emphasised her beautiful Negroid hair with natural twists and a little bleach, to stunning effect

3

Cosmetic hair treatments

About this chapter ...

In this chapter we look at the science behind the hair treatments that are used by people all over the world in order to enhance their appearance: styling, perming, and changing the colour of the hair.

From straightforward styling to elaborate perms, from a temporary tint to a platinum bleach, all these processes depend on changing part of the structure of hair. The stylists and technicians who have to apply them are expected to have a thorough understanding of hair structure, the hair growth cycle and the continuing care of hair. They need a working knowledge of the disorders of the hair and scalp, the chemistry of hair care products and the ways in which they protect the hair, and the science that underlies the various cosmetic procedures.

Just as a doctor takes a 'history' of a new patient in the surgery, so the stylist looks at the history of a client's hair and examines its condition, in particular whether there is evidence that it has been chemically treated previously. The doctor can only decide what can be done for the patient once that history is known and understood: in the same way, the most expert stylist can only decide what is or is not possible after that examination has been made.

Styling hair

Styling hair means temporarily or permanently altering its shape. We shall discuss perming in the next section. Here we are talking about the temporary changes brought about by setting the hair. Setting is different from perming in that

HAIR FACTS

Changing the hair

Whether your hair is straight or naturally curly depends on your genetic inheritance, which of course cannot be changed.

Any alteration to the natural state of hair must be brought about by either mechanical manipulation, or chemical change, or both.

there is no chemical reaction in the hair. All that happens is that some of the weak hydrogen bonds are broken by water and then re-form in the newly positioned hair as the water evaporates.

A curl can be produced by setting hair on a former such as a curler or roller – that is, allowing wet hair to dry while twisted round the former. (Fixing wet hair into pin curls has a similar effect.) After the curlers or rollers have been removed the hair holds its shape until it gets wet again.

In a perfect world, the hair could be left to dry naturally on the curlers or rollers and then combed out with a broad-toothed comb. But the pace and hurry of modern life makes this a luxury that we cannot afford, and some kind of hair dryer has to be used to speed the process up. Heat is a great enemy to hair, however, and that means that dryers must always be used with great care and on a moderate setting. A hair dryer on its hottest setting will reach temperatures well above that at which water boils. As we have seen, this can have a disastrous effect on the hair. Using a 'hot oil' has a protective effect. So too do hair mousses, which contain specially formulated resins.

Curls produced by setting are tight when they are first formed, but they can be brushed out into a lighter style. Using setting lotions or hair sprays gives a firmer effect, and helps to hold the temporary curl in for longer.

Softer, looser styles can be created by brushing and blow drying only, without using rollers. The principle is exactly the same as that of the setting process. The only difference is that the hydrogen bonds re-connect to form the style that has been shaped by the brush.

All hair gradually absorbs moisture from the air, and as the hydrogen bonds break it will in time lose its style – especially in damp weather!

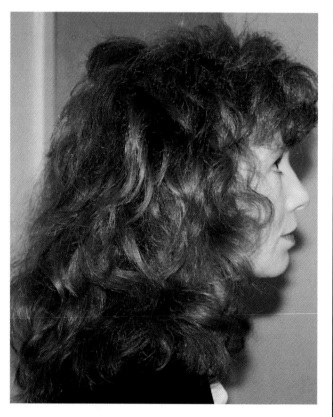

An excellent example of 'setting' to give a spectacular effect to already curly hair

---

HAIR FACTS

What happens during setting

First, read again the section in Chapter 1 of this book about the chemical structure of hair.

When hair is set, the millions of weak hydrogen bonds between the keratin chains in the hair are broken when the hair is wetted, and form up again in different places on the chains as the water evaporates during drying.

The strong disulphide linkages in hair can only be altered by chemical treatments, and are unaffected during setting. They keep the hair in its fundamental natural shape throughout repeated washing and drying.

Perming hair

The strong disulphide linkages in hair are formed when the hair cells harden into keratin in the hair follicle. These are the bonds that keep the hair shaft in shape. In order to change its shape, the disulphide bonds have to be broken down and re-formed into a different pattern. We saw that changes to hydrogen bonds in the setting process are only temporary. Chemical changes to the disulphide bonds are permanent.

The history of perms

People have been trying to turn straight hair into waves and curls for thousands of years. The women of Ancient Egypt used to apply a mixture of soil and water to their hair, wrap it on crudely made wooden 'rollers' and then bake the muddy mess in the sun – the results would have been anything but permanent, however! In fact, as we have seen, temporary waving is still carried out by setting damp or wet hair into a new shape on curlers or rollers. Heat from a dryer and the use of a setting lotion give a firmer, longer-lasting style. But the changes to the hair are the same as the Egyptian ladies brought about: only the weak hydrogen bonds in the hair are affected, and the hair goes back to its original shape as soon as it is dampened.

The first truly permanent waves became available in 1920. The waving lotion was

<u>Perming hair</u>

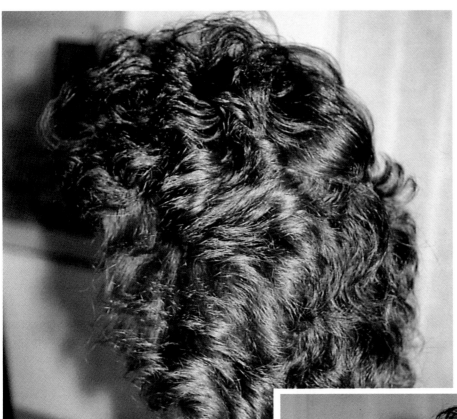

*A perfect example of hair which
has been given body and volume
by perming*

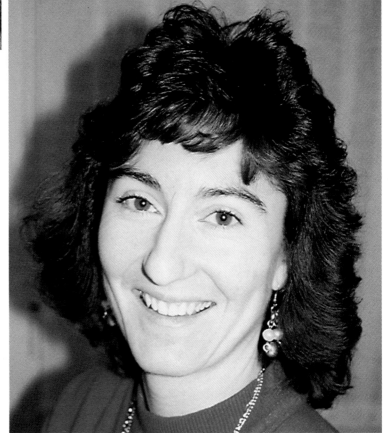

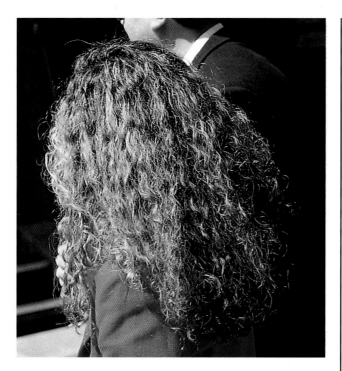

This permed and bleached long hair looks good at first glance, but the hair is dry and has no lustre

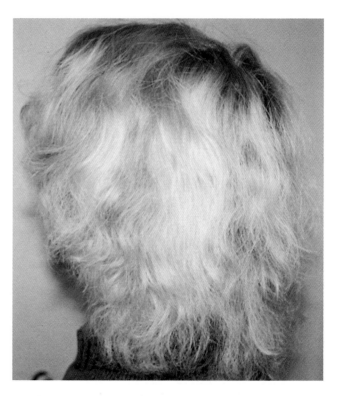

Dry, lifeless hair that has been repeatedly permed: the hair has also been bleached, and the darker roots are growing out in much better condition: at this stage it can no longer take a perm because virtually all the disulphide bonds have been broken

activated by heat from an electrical device. The early models did not have thermostats, and it was difficult to control their temperature. They had individual heaters for each curl, and clients found these heavy and uncomfortable. These early perms were harsh and drying, and left the hair in tight frizzy curls that were difficult to manage.

Early in the 1940s the 'cold wave' was introduced. This was basically the perming process that we use today. The cold wave had many advantages: the unpleasant heat and weight of the old appliances were completely eliminated, and the hair could be waved closer to the scalp.

Modern perms

A permanent wave is a process that creates a curl in the hair shaft by altering its internal chemical structure. This curl cannot be destroyed except by further chemical treatment.

A perm is not necessarily an easy option. Certainly, perming creates a style in the existing hair. But after perming the hair continues to grow as it did before, at the rate of a centimetre or so every month. The new hair, of course, grows straight. So the perm has to be either repeated or left to grow out. Some hair can stand up to repeated perming quite well, some can't!

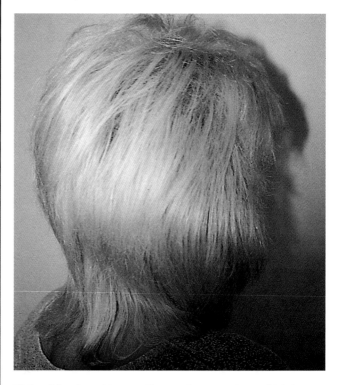

Hair with a long history of cosmetic processing, which is approaching the limit of its tolerance

Whether or not a perm will 'take' well depends on the basic nature of the hair, its past history of chemical treatments, if any, and the skill of the technician or stylist. Hair that has had a long history of perming, perhaps combined with tinting or bleaching, may have become so damaged as to be near the limit of what it will tolerate.

HAIR FACTS

pH and hair

The key to the perming process lies in the fact that perming solution is **alkaline**. What exactly does this mean in relation to hair?

When scientists talk to each other about alkaline solutions and acid solutions, they need a way of measuring alkalinity and acidity. The scale they use for their measurements is called the **pH scale**.

The pH scale ranges from pH 1 to pH 14. All you need to remember is that **acids** have pH numbers less than 7. **Alkalis** have pH numbers greater than 7. The more acid the solution, the lower is the pH number; the more alkaline the solution, the greater the pH number.

pH is measured using special **indicator papers** which change colour when the pH changes.

Hair responds to changes in pH. If a hair is placed in an alkaline solution it swells, and the scales of the cuticle lift. In a slightly acid solution, the scales lie smoothly and the hair is soft. In a strongly acid or alkaline solution, however, the keratin protein starts to break down.

The perming process

The hair is first washed and then wound on to some kind of former, such as a curler or a rod. The perm lotion is applied to the hair. Because the lotion is alkaline (pH about 9) the scales of the cuticle open slightly, allowing the lotion to flow under the cuticle and into the cortex. Here it reacts with the keratin of the cortex, breaking some of the disulphide cross-links within and between the protein chains. The hair swells and 'softens', so that it can stretch to take up the shape of the formers.

After a while the perm lotion is thoroughly rinsed away and a **neutralising lotion** is applied. This re-forms the broken cross-links, which makes the hair harden into its new, curlier shape. This stage is the key to a successful perm: failure to rinse and neutralise properly can lead to many problems, including scalp irritation and damage to the structure of the hair shaft.

HAIR FACTS

What happens during perming

Today's 'cold' permanent wave lotions contain substances called **reducing agents**, in an alkaline solution. The reducing agent most often used is called **ammonium thioglycollate**. Reducing agents act on the keratin in the hair, breaking the disulphide linkages that join the pairs of cysteine units together. The result is that the keratin softens and swells. The softened hair is then put into its new shape. As it is manipulated the cysteine linkages slip past each other and realign themselves with new cysteine partners (see page 91).

Neutralising lotion is then applied. This contains **oxidising agents**. One that is often used is **hydrogen peroxide**, the same substance that is used in hair bleaches. Oxidising agents work in the opposite way to reducing agents. They make the cysteine units link together into pairs again, hardening the hair and giving it its new, permanent shape.

In hair that has been repeatedly permed the original disulphide cross-links may have been broken and re-formed so many times that hardly any remain.

In order to illustrate the process of permanent waving, we will follow a client through the full procedure.

This client, like many others, wants her hair put into a manageable style, with curl and body. It is vital that the stylist understands the past history of her hair. It is permed every three or four months, and tinted more frequently. Fortunately her hair is naturally very resilient, and has not suffered unduly. In expert hands, a perm should be straightforward.

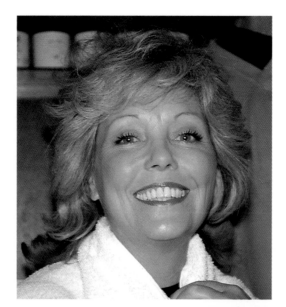

The client ready for the perm

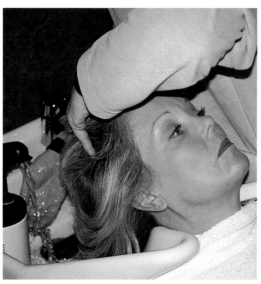

Shampooing at the basin

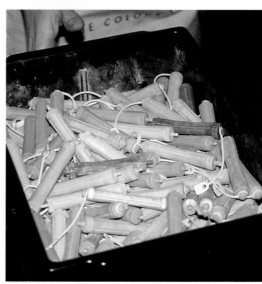

Rollers of various sizes ready for use

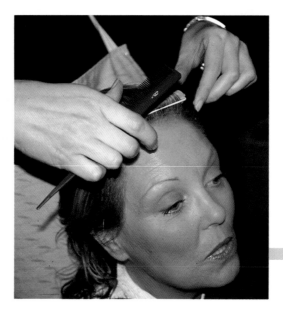

Putting in the first roller …

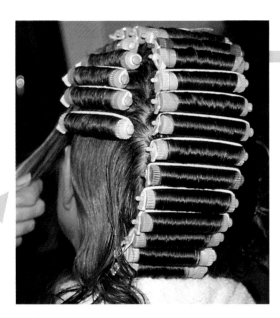

... almost done!

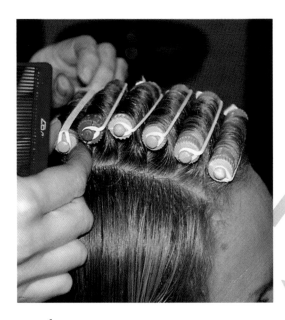

... and more ...

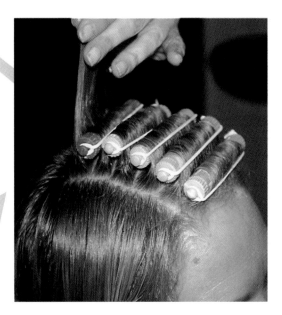

... still more ...

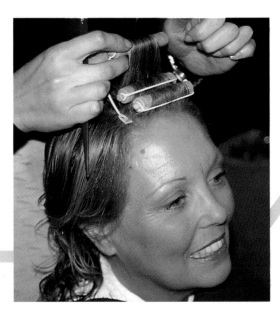

... then more ...

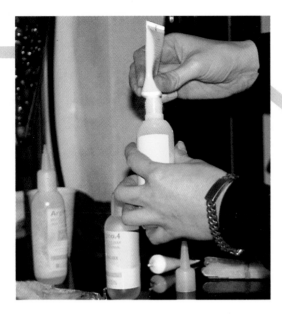

Preparing the perming solution …

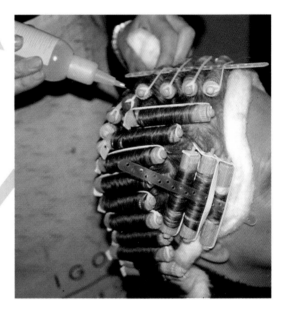

… and applying it …

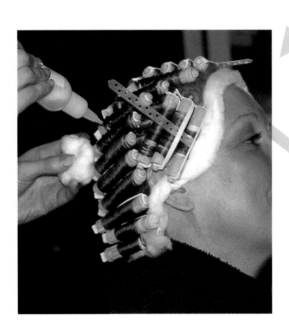

… evenly …

For the purposes of photography, the technician has removed her gloves. Under normal circumstances gloves should always be worn when working with chemicals.

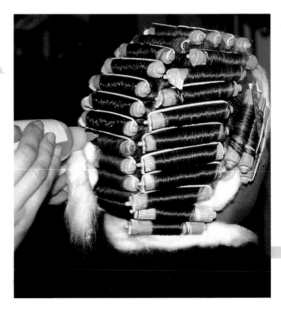

… and systematically …

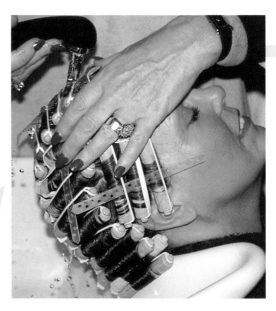

Thorough rinsing of the perming solution – best done using the backwash

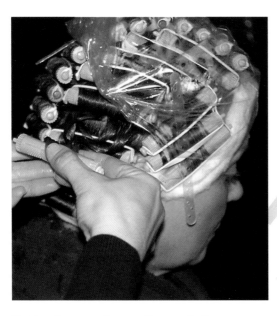

Testing the perm: is more time needed?

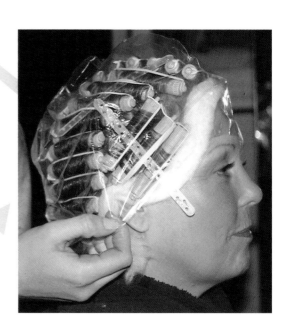

Perming is complete

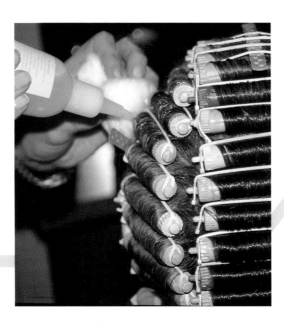

... and thoroughly

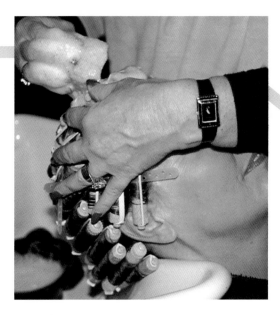

Neutralising the perm

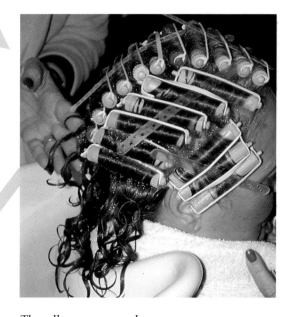

The rollers are removed

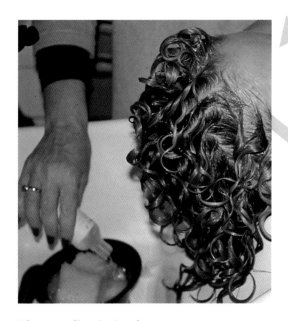

The neutraliser is rinsed away

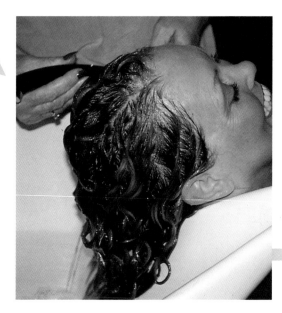

Care is taken to avoid tangling

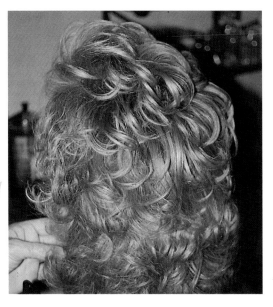

Nearly there!

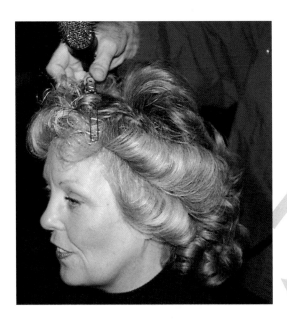

Putting the finishing touches

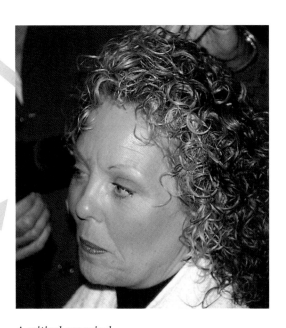

A critical appraisal ...

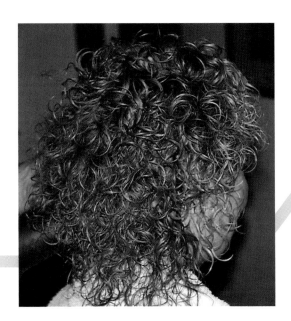

Ready for blow drying and styling

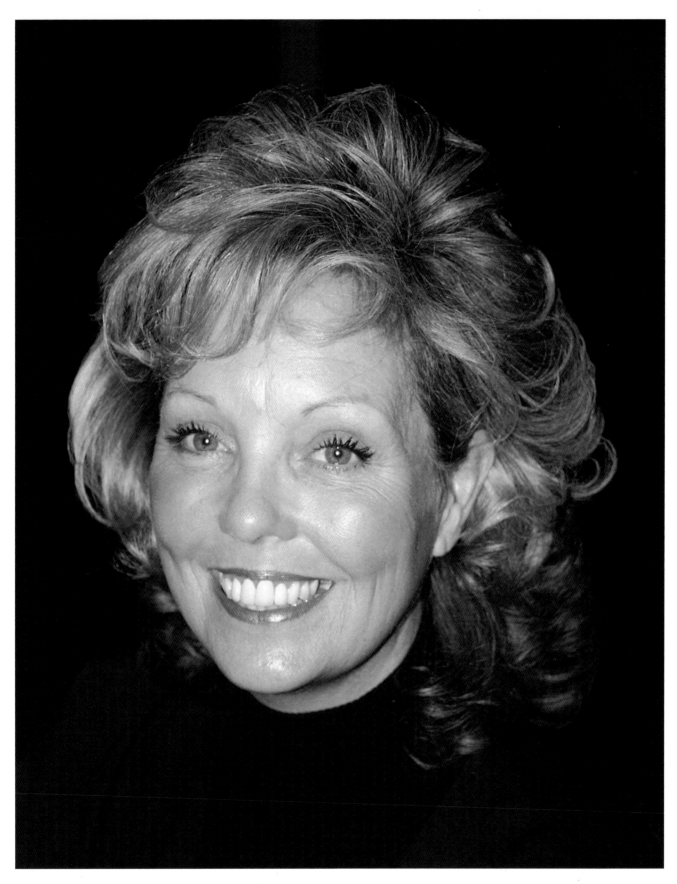

A successful perm, and a delighted client

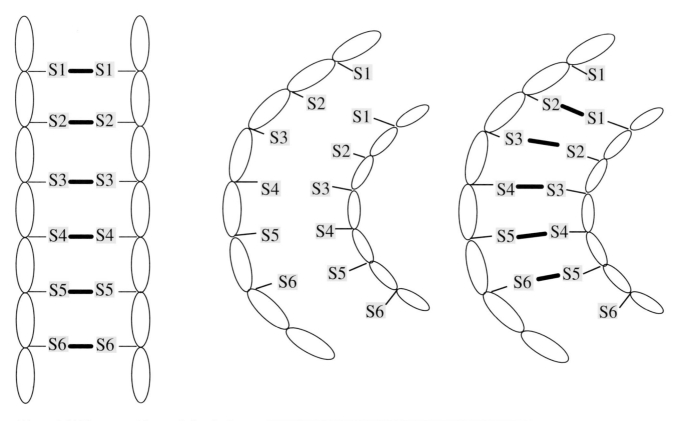

(Above, left) The normal internal chemical structure of the hair protein, showing unbroken disulphide bonds; (centre) in perming, bonds in the hair wrapped around a roller are broken by a reducing agent; (right) after oxidation the bonds are re-aligned in a different order, permanently changing the shape and producing a curl

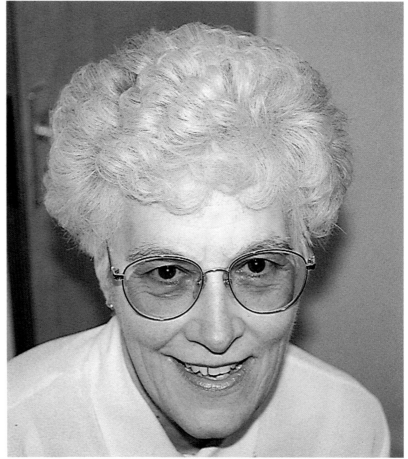

Many people decide on a perm as they get older and their hair length and density diminishes: perming gives volume and – as seen on the right – is not necessarily excessive or obviously damaging

Some people's hair is resistant to the chemicals used to open and close the scales of the cuticle. Often this is an inherited tendency. The only way to deal with it is to use stronger chemicals. Great care is needed with these, however, as they may damage the hair shaft so severely that it breaks.

Red hair is an example of this. The keratin of red hair tends to contain more sulphur than usual – it can be twice as much as the average – because it contains a high proportion of cysteine units. That means that there are many more disulphide linkages to be broken, and it is therefore more likely that a perm will fail to 'take' on red hair.

Perm shock

Once the perming solution has been put on, the hair is in a very vulnerable condition. The keratin is softened and greatly swollen, particularly during rinsing, the cortex is in the process of being chemically changed, and the cuticle may have been slightly damaged. At this point every possible care is needed to protect the hair from any unwanted change in conditions.

For example, sudden temperature changes can damage the softened keratin to such an extent that the hair may break down completely. A story is told about a Swedish lady who was having a perm one winter's day. The temperature outside was well below freezing, although in the warm salon it was around 22 °C. The perming solution had already been applied when suddenly the lady glimpsed in the mirror a friend of hers walking by in the street. Impulsively, she rushed outside to greet her. The horrified hairdresser had to chase after her and bring her back indoors, where she set to work to try to re-equilibrate her client's head by wrapping hot towels around it to get the temperature back up again.

After perming

Even though the perming process seems complete when the client has left the salon, the hair continues to form new bonds for two or three days. It is important that the hair should *not* be shampooed during those few days: shampooing may interrupt this 'curing' process and spoil the carefully constructed curls, or even lead to hair breakage.

Moreover, if the perm has not been neutralised completely, using a shampoo (whatever the brand) may cause the perm to fail disastrously. This is not the shampoo's fault, nor is it the client's.

It is wise to advise a client, however thrilled she may be with her newly permed hair, that her hair needs conditioning regularly, especially thoroughly, and very frequently.

HAIR FACTS

Skin: acid and alkaline

After any hair care procedure, we need to consider how the skin is left, and in particular how acid or alkaline it is.

The pH of the surface of normal skin is between 5 and 6. That is, it is slightly acid. This is often referred to as the skin's 'acid mantle', but this is more of an emotional than a strictly scientific statement. The acidity is due in part to the sebum, the natural oil produced by the skin, which is itself slightly acid.

One important function of the skin is to protect the tissues lying beneath it. The skin does this by acting as a barrier, regulating liquid loss from inside and keeping excess liquid outside the body.

It also protects the body from infection. The acidity of the skin surface slows down the growth of bacteria and makes it harder for them to enter the body. If the acidity of the skin is affected – if the pH rises above 5–6, say – infections are more likely. This can happen if the pH is not adjusted after chemical hairdressing processes such as perming, by very thorough rinsing and careful neutralisation.

Relaxing (straightening) hair

Relaxing is the opposite of perming. It is traditionally used by people with Afro-Caribbean hair to straighten their hair. It is popular because it makes hair easier to manage.

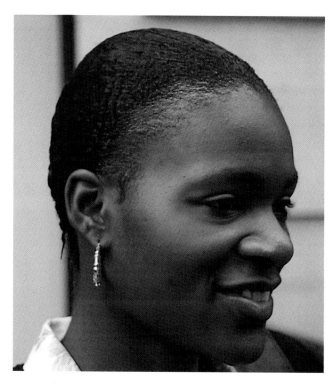

This lady's hair has been gently relaxed

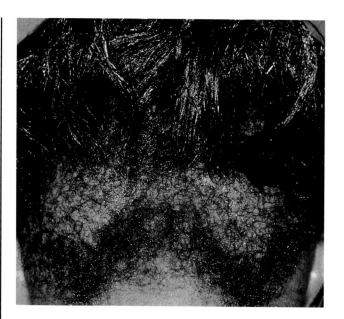

Hair breakage at the back of the neck associated with relaxing and traction

The chemistry of the relaxing process is identical with that of perming, with the breaking of disulphide linkages and re-forming of the hair shape (in a straighter arrangement this time, rather than in curls), followed by re-making of the linkages.

The oval (elliptical) shape and natural crimp of Afro-Caribbean hair makes it difficult to straighten without damage. The chemical treatment can weaken the hair structure, and breakage after relaxation treatment is not uncommon. Contributing factors include incorrect concentrations of relaxing solution, mistakes in timing the application, and incomplete rinsing. Often the hair breakage is seen at the back of the neck. In addition, straightening leaves the hair fibres in a high degree of torsional stress (twisting), and a slightly wavy look. This makes them liable to rapid weathering, with the cuticle wearing down at the ends of the cross-sectional ellipse and a characteristic lengthwise splitting.

Perming different types of hair

Fine Caucasoid hair is probably the 'worst' hair to try to perm. It has the smallest diameter, and needs the minimum amount of perming

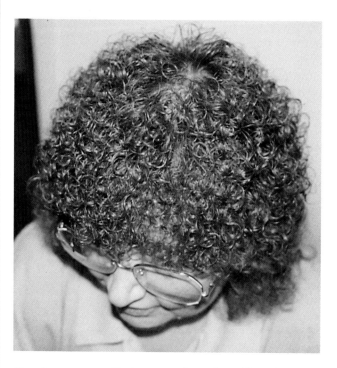

Grossly over-permed hair: repeated perming will produce dry, damaged hair unless very expertly performed

solution and processing time. The photograph above shows you what the results of over-perming can be!

Strong, dark Caucasoid hair will take a perm reasonably well, even when tightly wound formers are not used.

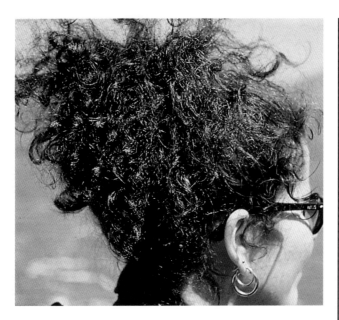

No comment needed!

Problems in perming and straightening

In some countries, up to 70% of women have permed hair, in order to give their hair curl and body. In expert hands, perming can create wonderful effects. And it is a tribute to the skill of stylists and technicians that so many perms are successful and attractive, despite all the complexity of the chemistry and science of perming. The disasters that occasionally result from the efforts of amateurs can be all too obvious.

Unfortunately, not all hair is suitable for perming – and so many clients with thinning hair seem to want a perm! – let alone the delicate question of whether the style that has charmed the client will in fact suit her. The table below shows some problems that can arise with perming.

■ Although some of the disulphide linkages re-form during neutralisation, a proportion fail to do so and remain broken. The hair is thereby weakened.

■ Where the cuticle scales fail to close up tightly again after perming, the hair is left with a roughened surface and weathers more quickly.

■ Incorrect application of perming, straightening or relaxing solutions can dissolve the hair fibres or lead to breakage, usually quite close to the scalp. This kind of breakage almost never happens on the same day as perming. It is believed to be the result of either over-perming or poor neutralisation.

Changing hair colour

If ever there was a mark of our desire to change the way other people see us, changing hair colour has to be it! For example, for thousands of years Indian ladies have put red highlights into their dark hair using pure henna, a semi-permanent dye prepared from the Egyptian privet (*Lawsonia inermis*), a flowering shrub that grows in their country.

Permanent waving process variability: the factors to be considered before perming

Hair stock	Hair type	Hair history	Perm process			Post perm
			Reduction	Rinse	Neutralise	
Caucasian	Dry	Perm	Chemistry	Time	Chemistry	Advise
– Northern Europe	Greasy	Colour	– acid		– age of product	
– Latin	Normal	Bleach	– alkaline	Temperature	– concentration	Warm water
– Indian	Mixed	Weathered	– age of product		– temperature of solution	
Asian			– concentration	Volume	– ambient temperature	Perm type/style
– Chinese	Curly	Normal	– temperature of solution		– time to apply	
– Japanese	Straight	Mixed	– ambient temperature		– time to work	Product use
			– time to apply		– pre-wet	
	Long		– time to work		– post-wet	Activity
African	Short		– pre-wet		– solution:hair mass ratio	
			– post-wet			
	Thick		– solution:hair mass ratio			
	Thin					
			Curlers			
	Coarse		– size			
	Medium		– type			
	Fine		Hair tension			

Changing hair colour

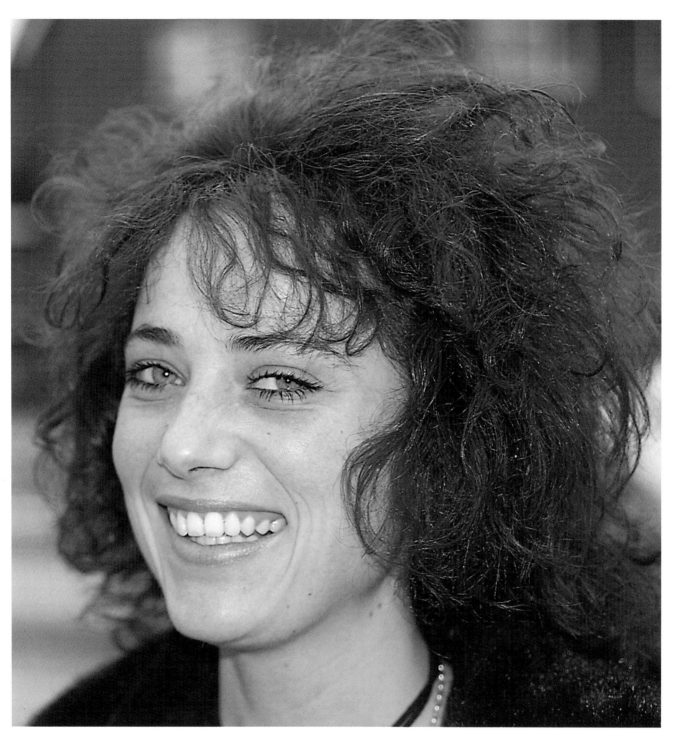

Changing your hair colour is exciting, but take care – it doesn't always turn out exactly as you expected! Understanding the colour circle is important (see page 97)

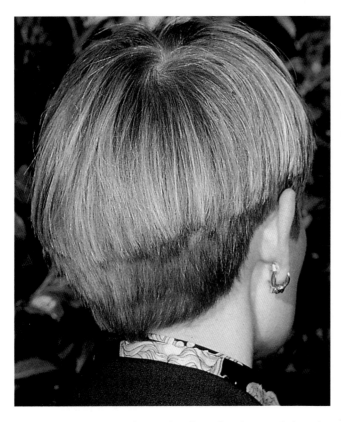

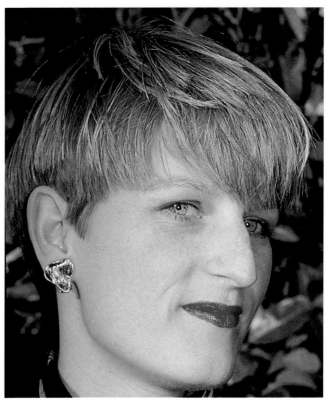

A clever stylist who understands colour chemistry and the colour circle can produce excellent tinting in keeping with the client's expectations: this, together with regular styling, produces a satisfied client

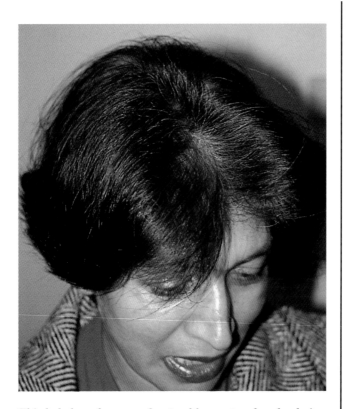

This lady has always used natural henna to colour her hair

Colour of every kind is a feature of all our lives. We particularly value the colour of our hair. We may perhaps quickly pull out the first grey hairs that we notice – but we all know that will not be the end of the matter. Once the hair follicle has stopped producing pigment cells, it is highly unlikely to start again. The 'new' hair will be grey too.

Hair colour is due to the present of melanin pigments in the cortex of the hair shaft. As we have seen there are two kinds of pigment, eumelanin and phaeomelanin. The cuticle is colourless and translucent: it looks like a polythene sheath. The colour we see is due to a combination of light that has passed through the coloured cortex and light that is reflected by the smooth cuticle. If there is no pigment in the cortex, the hair looks white.

The colour of hair can be changed in only three ways:

- it can be made lighter, either wholly or in part
- it can be made darker, either wholly or in part
- it can be changed to an entirely different shade, either wholly or in part.

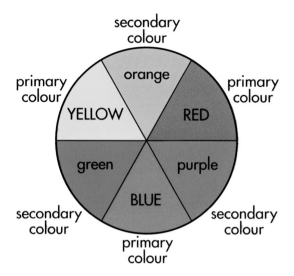

The colour circle

You probably learnt at school that sunlight is made up of light of many different colours. You may perhaps have seen those colours in the glittering flashes of light that sparkle in a diamond. A more everyday sighting is in a rainbow. In a bright rainbow you can clearly make out the separate colours arranged in order, with red on the outside and violet on the inside of the arc. This array of colours is called the **spectrum**. In the spectrum of sunlight, colours that are similar to each other – red and orange, for example – are seen side by side, and blend together.

Colour scientists have a special way of viewing the spectrum. The colours are arranged in a circle, in the way shown here. In this **colour circle** similar colours are still placed side by side, but they are separated from each other.

There are three basic or **primary colours**: red, yellow and blue. These are spaced equally around the colour circle. In between them are the colours made by combining the primary colours together in pairs: these are called **combination colours**. Orange is produced by combining red and yellow, green by combining yellow and blue, and violet by combining blue and red. Yellow, orange and red are often seen as 'warm' colours, and violet, blue and green as 'cold' colours.

All the combination colours come in different **shades**: for instance, you get a reddish orange if there is more red than yellow in the mixture, and yellowish orange if there is more yellow than red. The exact shade depends on the proportions of the colours in the mixture.

In the colour circle, each of the primary colours lies opposite a combination colour: red lies opposite green, orange lies opposite blue, purple lies opposite yellow. These pairs of 'opposite' colours are called **complementary colours**. If you mix red and green, you get neither red nor green but a greyish colour. The same applies with the other complementary pairs. They cancel each other out when they are mixed.

It can be extremely useful to understand this effect when you are colouring hair. Suppose a client's hair has an orange tinge after bleaching: colouring lightly with the complementary colour blue will cancel out the unwanted orange. Similarly if hair has an unpleasantly yellowish look, tinting with the complementary colour violet may provide a solution.

Some interesting results are seen when more than two colours are mixed. A mixture of red and violet looks brown. Suppose we add a little yellow: the yellow and violet produce grey, and the result is a softer, more mousy brown. Add a little red instead, and you may get a chestnut colour. Mixing red, yellow and purple together will give black, or at least a very dark grey.

In the practical world, the six colours of the spectrum are not enough to meet all our needs in hair colouring. But hair colour manufacturers can get any colour a client might choose by the careful mixing of these six, plus black and white, in various proportions.

Colouring hair

Colour agents

Colouring agents for hair are of four main types: temporary hair colour, natural colourings, semi-permanent dyes and permanent dyes.

Temporary hair colour

The dyes used as temporary hair colouring agents were originally developed for use in textile industry. They are acidic dyes that are deposited on the outside of the hair, so they do not penetrate the hair shaft. They affect the way in which the cuticle reflects light, and they tend to make the hair look flat. They are easily shampooed off the hair, so they last through only a few washes. They are available as rinses, gels, mousses and sprays.

Unlike some of the permanent hair dyes, temporary hair colours carry very little risk of irritant or allergic dermatitis when they are used.

Natural colourings

Natural colours have been used on hair since ancient times. Most of them are made from plants. Henna is by far the best known. It is widely used to this day to redden hair, especially dark hair, and the colour produced lasts through several shampoos. But its concentration is difficult to control, and hence results can be unpredictable. It has been reported to cause asthma and allergies in some people, and people who suffer from these ailments should be wary of using it.

Henna should not be used on grey hair, as it turns it orange!

Semi-permanent dyes

Special hair dye preparations are made for colouring grey hair. They can be used to add highlights too. They do not contain a single dye but mixtures of red, yellow, blue, and orange dyes in various proportions. The dyes have small molecules, which means they can pass through the cuticle into the cortex easily, and

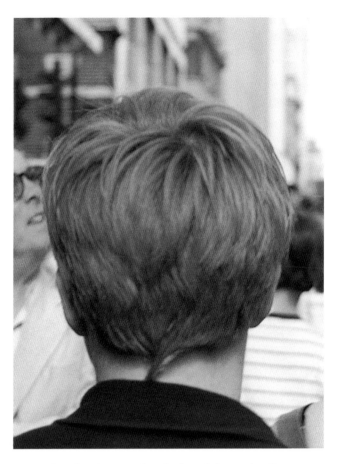

Here colour has been used to fresh and dramatic effect

without damaging the scales of the cuticle. Since they can enter the hair shaft easily, they can also be washed out relatively easily.

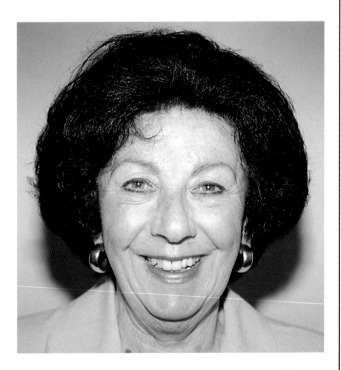

This lady has coloured her hair for many years: careful treatment and her technician's expert skill have concealed the premature greying she disliked

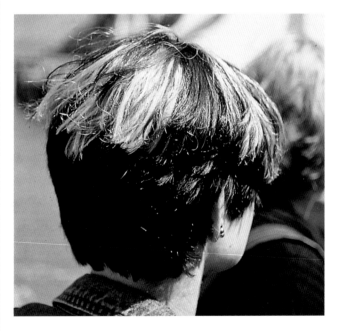

The result of inexpert colouring

They can last for 6–12 weeks, and tend to fade or lighten over this time. The red dyes seem to be the quickest to leak out of the hair, and as a result the hair can look drab after a few washes.

Semi-permanent dye preparations do not contain bleaches, and are therefore safe to use. They can be used at home. Without bleach, however, they cannot colour hair lighter than its natural shade.

Lightening hair

Hair is made lighter by changing part or all of the melanin pigment in the cortex into a colourless substance. The melanin is not washed out of the hair – it is changed chemically, and the change cannot be reversed.

The chemical solutions used are called **bleaches**. They contain oxidising agents, like those in neutralising lotions for perms, in alkaline solution. The bleach most commonly used is hydrogen peroxide. Hydrogen peroxide can be used alone to lighten dark hair, or together with a colouring agent (a **tint**).

As you will recall, red and blond hair contains more phaeomelanin than eumelanin. On the other hand, dark hair – black or dark brown – contains more eumelanin than phaeomelanin. Of the two kinds of melanin in hair, eumelanin is the more easily removed from the cortex by bleaches. This is why bleached dark hair tends to look reddish: the eumelanin has been decolorised, and what is left is mostly phaeomelanin. Further bleaching removes the phaeomelanin too. This is also why red hair is harder to bleach than dark hair.

Strongly bleached hair looks yellowish, because keratin itself is naturally pale yellow. This natural colour is the reason why an elderly person's white hair looks slightly yellow at the roots, as mentioned in Chapter 1. It also explains why repeatedly bleached hair looks the colour of nicotine-stained skin. It needs to be tinted as well as bleached if it is to be turned white or a 'platinum' blond.

The stages of lightening hair
The colour of hair changes as it is lightened, as more and more eumelanin and then phaeomelanin is removed step by step.

Suppose that a black-haired client decides she would like to be a platinum blonde. To make this change at a single session, her stylist would

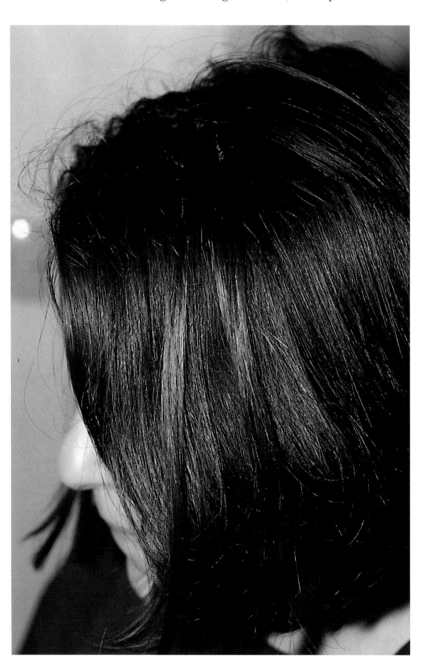

The eumelanin has been removed more easily than the phaeomelanin from this dark hair, hence the parti-coloured appearance

have to use the most powerful bleaching chemicals available. They would certainly damage her hair to a marked extent. It would be less damaging to carry out the process in several stages – up to a dozen, perhaps. During that time her hair would change from black to red, and then lighten gradually from red to orange, orange to yellow, and finally from yellow to white. Some of the stages might well have to be repeated.

The stylist might decide that a three-step or five-step programme would be possible, changing first from black to red, then from red to yellow, and finally to white. What has to be considered before any final decision is taken is how to keep damage to the cuticle to a minimum, and above all what will be the final effect of the programme on the quality of the hair.

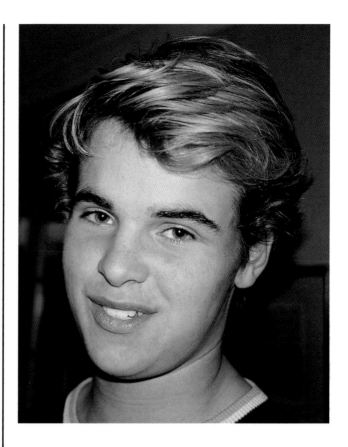

HAIR FACTS

How lightening works

The oxidising agents in bleaches take part in a chemical reaction with melanin. They provide the melanin molecule with oxygen from their own molecules. The oxidised melanin molecule is colourless.

Melanin is contained in the cortex of the hair. For the oxidising agent to reach the melanin, therefore, it has to get through the cuticle. In the alkaline solution of the bleach formulation, the scales of the cuticle are raised and the bleach chemicals can then penetrate the cortex.

Problems in the bleaching process
Raising the scales of the cuticle for penetration by the bleach is in itself a potentially risky process, and one that should only be carried out by a knowledgeable stylist or technician. *Repeated* bleaching can leave permanently raised scales and upset the moisture content. It increases the porosity of the hair, and this makes further bleaching more difficult: very porous hair bleaches badly, with uneven shading. Repeated bleaching leaves weak, brittle hairs which have little shine or lustre, and which weather rapidly. Additional cosmetic procedures such as perming simply make things worse.

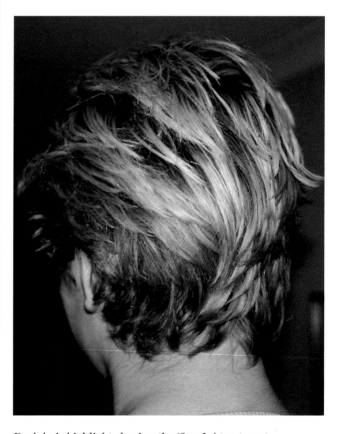

Dark hair highlighted using the 'Sun In' treatment

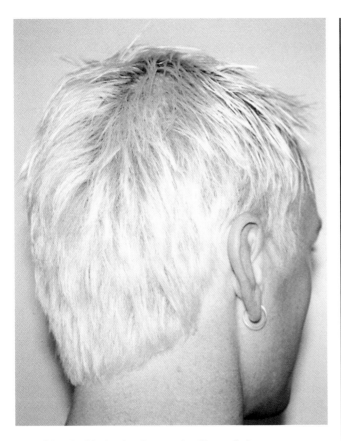

Over-bleached hair: the damage is all too obvious

Bleaching is not the only effect of treating hair with oxidising agents. Side-reactions often happen, such as breakage of some of the strong disulphide bonds of the hair. Re-bleaching, which means treating the whole length of the hair rather than just the roots, is certain to break more of these.

The cuticle is especially easily weakened in this way. As a result it becomes extremely easy to strip it away from the cortex, even during routine hair care. Wet combing, for instance, becomes more difficult and causes additional damage. Backcombing is especially damaging because it can removes large amounts of cuticle with a single sweep of the comb.

Bleached hair, being porous, swells more readily when it is wet, and its wet strength is reduced still further. Eventually the hair protein may become so weakened that it separates and the hair breaks.

Permanent hair colour

This is the kind of hair colouring that is used most commonly throughout the world. It is the type that has to be used if a complete change of hair colour is required. Highlighting or colouring just part of the hair using a permanent colour is possible, however.

When changing hair colour, it is wise not to make a permanent change of colour all at once, especially if the new colour will be very different from the old. It is sensible to try a temporary colour first: this can be washed out straight away if the effect is disappointing. The next step would be to use a semi-permanent dye. Only if this is successful would it be advisable to move to permanent colouring, and that is something that should ideally be done by a professional.

The **two-step** colouring process starts by stripping the hair of all the melanin that gives it its natural colour. Hydrogen peroxide in 30–40% solution is used. This is one of the harshest of all procedures used on hair, because the bleach destroys hair keratin. The hair can look lifeless when bleaching is complete, and another chemical process follows, using a new colour.

A more typical procedure uses a gentler bleach (20% hydrogen peroxide solution) together with a dye and an alkaline soap or synthetic cleansing agent.

Allergies have been reported after the use of permanent colours, especially preparations containing the chemical ammonium persulphate. It is *always* wise to carry out a patch test on a client's skin before using any colouring process, in case there is any possibility of irritating, unsightly or painful allergy following the treatment. No colouring agent should ever be used on a client who is showing clear signs of dermatitis.

When shampooing after hair colouring, or indeed after any chemical processing of hair, use a shampoo with an acid balance as this will help the cuticle scales to close up and lie smooth again.

With regular professional re-tinting, using the same product, the hair can be kept the same colour for as long as required.

The colouring process step by step

This client's hair has been growing for about six years to reach this length. It has not been chemically treated before. It is in good condition, with good shine, but not a great deal of fullness or body.

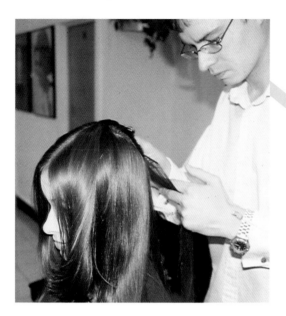

The stylist discusses the appropriate style for this client's hair: it is decided to follow the natural fall of the hair and the client's jawline

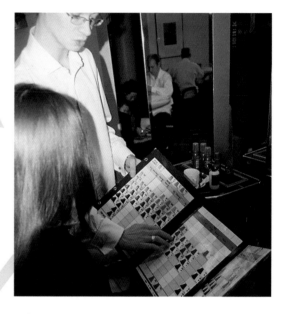

Selecting the colour: it is decided to lighten individual hair shafts with synthetic permanent dyes designed to complement the client's natural dark brown shade ('lowlighting') – lightening the hair too much would require heavy bleaching and might spoil its lustre

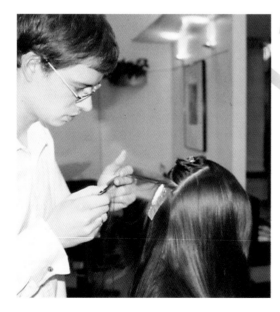

The process involves applying mixtures of dyes with hydrogen peroxide layer by layer to the hair

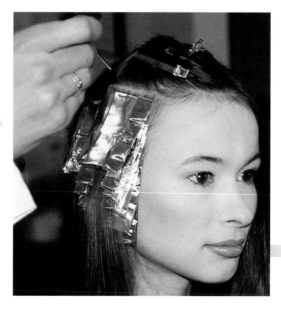

Foil is used to separate the layers of hair

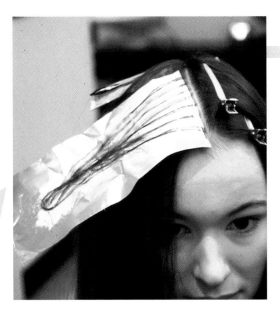

How the foil protects the untreated hair

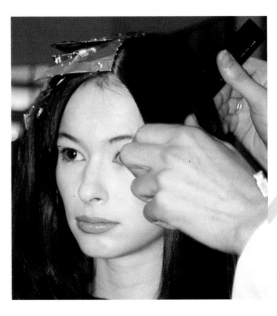

… and meticulous care!

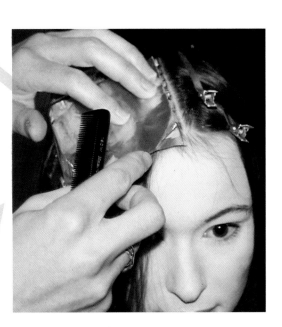

… and patient, unhurried working …

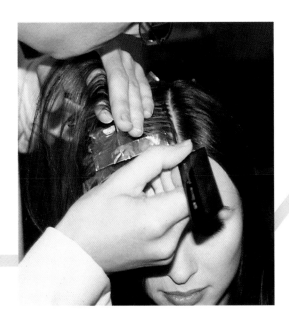

To get the desired effect requires systematic application …

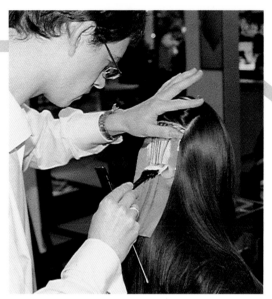

The application continues ...

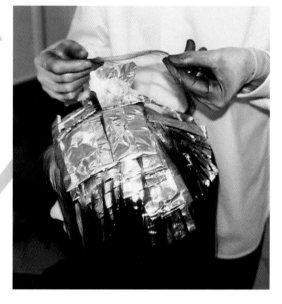

... almost done ...

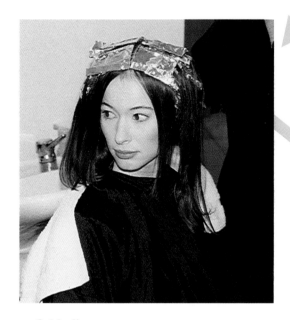

... finished!

Heat is applied to complete the process: the heat raises the cuticle and allows the colouring solution to penetrate the cortex more quickly

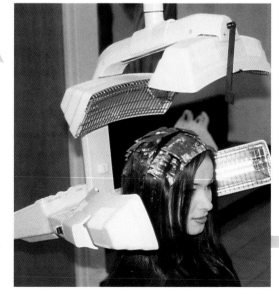

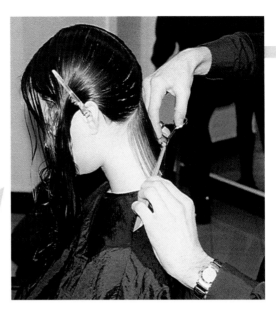

Using high-quality scissors ensures a clean cut

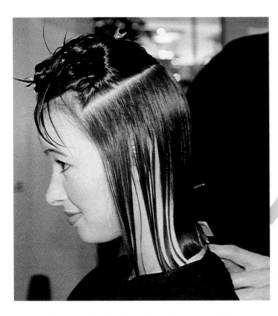

… and cut ready for the client's chosen style

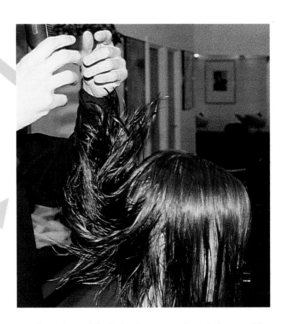

… the coloured hair is shampooed and thoroughly rinsed …

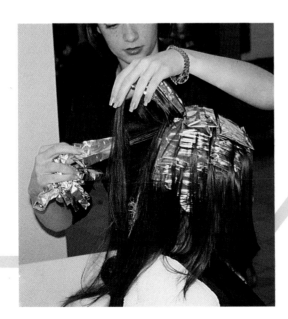

The foil is removed …

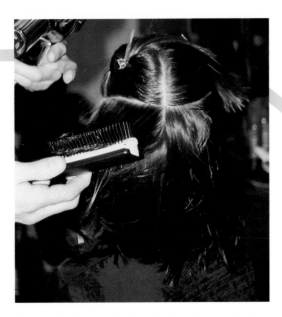

Drying the hair, using low heat and a rounded brush

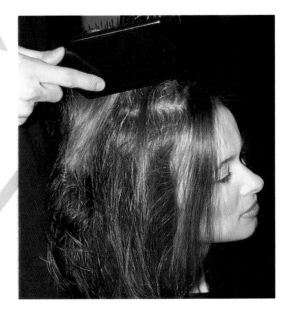

The style takes shape ...

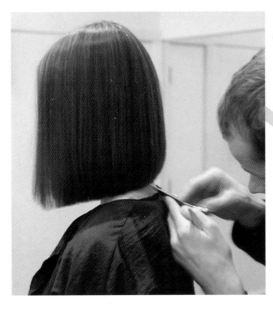

... it's nearly complete

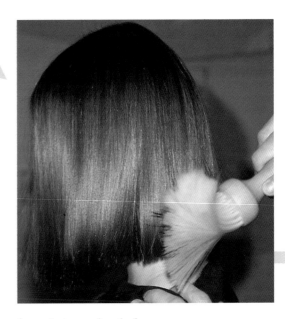

Loose hairs are brushed away

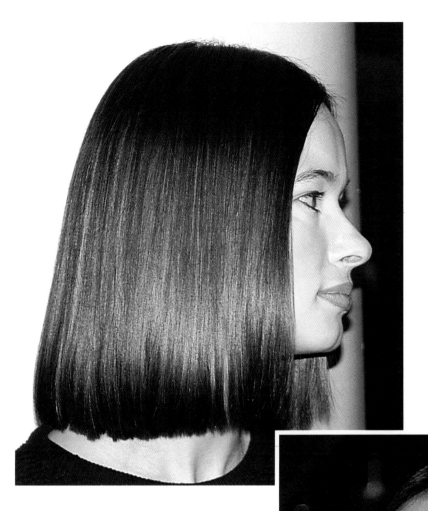

A satisfied – and transformed – client!

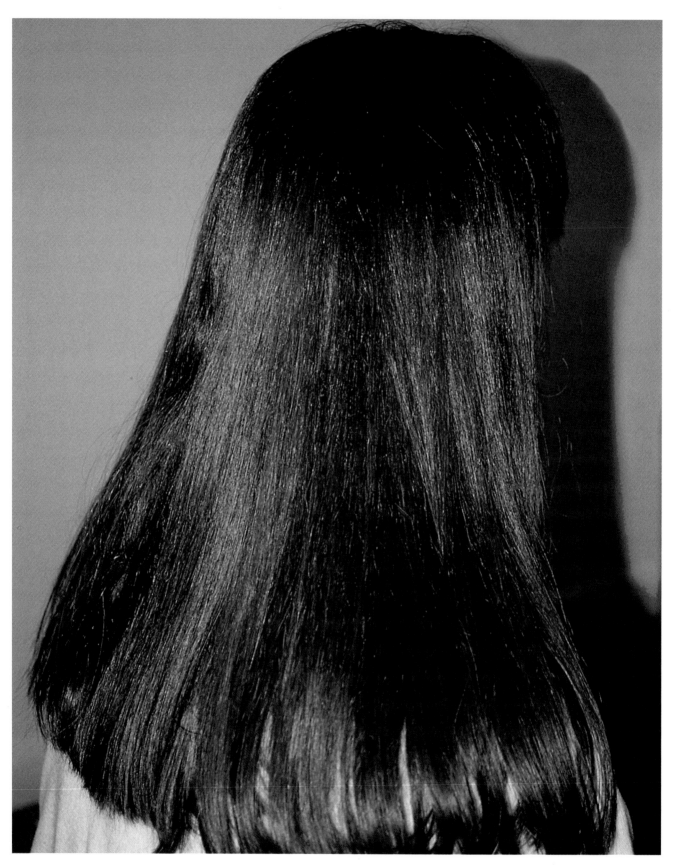

Why doesn't all hair look as good as this? No heat has ever been used on this lady's hair: like many others in the Far East she always lets it dry naturally after shampooing. She uses a very broad-toothed comb and has never processed her hair

Cosmetic problems

About this chapter ...

In this chapter we look at a few common problematic conditions that are met with in the hair salon. We explore the basic changes that can happen and the reasons for them, and we look at their appearance when viewed under the microscope.

Most of these changes are difficult if not impossible to reverse, although a skilled hairdresser will know whether there are any useful repair measures that might be taken. All could have been prevented, however, if simple precautions had been taken.

Fortunately, cosmetic disasters are fairly rare, so this is a short chapter!

This is how we think healthy hair should look: long, luxuriant and shining. All too often, however, people find their own hair falls short of the ideal. And many of them lay the responsibility for all their hair problems on the last product they put on their hair.

But the hair's history goes back much further than that. A scientific understanding of hair can help us to read 'the record of the hair'. This may well help us to identify any cosmetic or even medical problems.

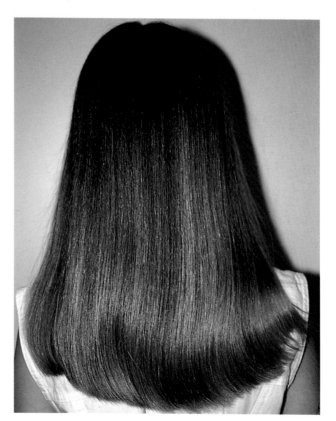

Care and attention based on good hair 'science' ensures beautiful, lustrous hair

Green hair

This condition is always associated with copper in some form and tends to affect repeatedly bleached hair. It is never seen in black hair, as the green becomes lost in the background colour. It may come from swimming pool water, especially where chloride treatment or copper algicides are used. Interestingly, it may be the result of high levels of copper in pipes in the home. This may have come from the water company's treatment plant, or from new copper piping in the house. In a house that has both old iron water pipes and new copper ones, there may be hugely increased copper levels in the drinking water. Green hair can even follow a good long soak in a bath that has been cleaned with old bathroom cleaners containing high chloride levels! And just occasionally it is the result of using a bleach.

Using a lemon juice rinse may improve the colour. There are commercial products that can help: an experienced hair stylist can advise on which might be used.

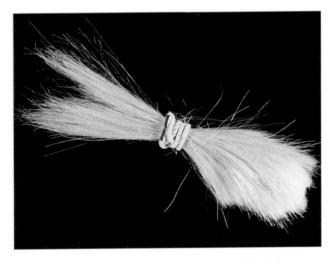

A classical case of green hair: this is seen in light hair, often hair that has been bleached

Bubble hair

People will tell you that their bubble hair 'just happened', quite suddenly, after they had been doing the same things to their hair for a long time. Then all at once they noticed tiny 'bubbles' in the ends of their hair.

Invariably, bubble hair is caused by some kind of heating appliance, most often curling irons.

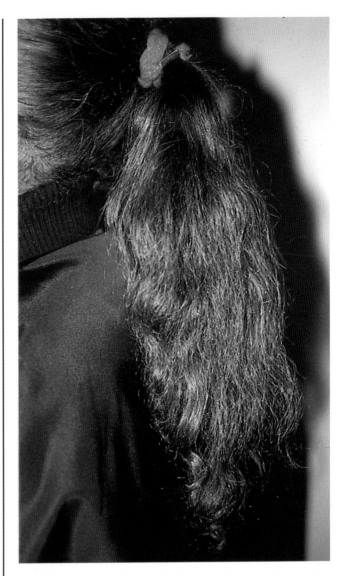

Hair that has been damaged by heat, perhaps by drying with a hair dryer on too high a setting

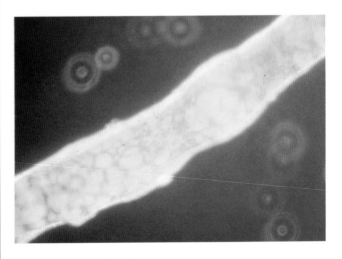

A classical case of bubble hair

These operate somewhere between 120 and 180 °C, roughly speaking. Water boils at 100 °C. If a hot curling iron is put on to wet hair, it boils the water inside the hair. The boiling water softens the keratin of the cortex; then the steam from the boiling water expands and forms tiny bubbles inside the hair. Eventually the hair breaks off, either at or somewhere near a bubble.

Every woman who has used curling irons knows that they work better on some days than others. One day she may have them just a little hotter than usual: that might be just enough to cause bubble hair, and for the affected hair to break off.

Although the sufferer usually claims that her hair was perfectly normal until she changed the hair product she was using, further enquiry always uncovers a history of increased or excessive cosmetic treatments. Usually bubble hair happens to people who are doing a lot of styling to their hair at home. And it is always, always associated with the use of heated appliances on damp hair.

Hair spray accumulation

This photograph was – quite wrongly – diagnosed as head lice!

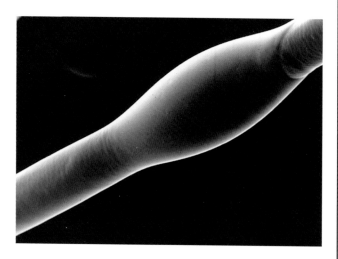

An electronmicrograph of a droplet of hair spray

In fact it shows a droplet of hair spray which has dried on a single hair forming a perfectly smooth cylinder around it. It has not touched another hair at all.

This photograph shows a hair spray droplet on hairs that are touching each other. There is one hair running this way —— and another one here. The spray has 'welded' the two together.

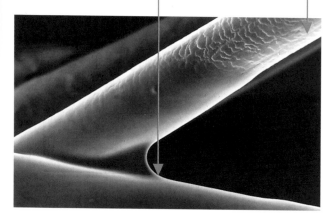

A spot weld between two hairs produced by a droplet of a modern hair spray

In this photo you can see a perfect replica of the cuticle of the second hair, here.

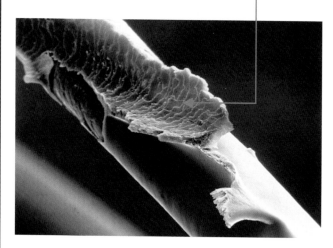

This kind of replica may be seen in heavily sprayed hair which is not washed often enough

What has happened here was that the lady concerned was washing her hair about once a week, and applying hair spray frequently and generously between shampoos. By the end of each week, significant amounts of hair spray had built up on her hair. Fortunately, modern shampoo technology is excellent at removing even a week's accumulation of hair spray, grease and dirt.

Matting and tangling: bird's nest hair

Tangled hair is very common. It is made worse by combing or brushing wet hair, since there is always more friction in wet hair because water raises the cuticle scales.

'Bird's nest hair' is the vivid term used to describe hair that has all at once become a severely tangled mat. One very bad attack of this kind happened to a lady with long black hair whose religion forbade her to treat her hair cosmetically in any way. She had just used a conditioning product on it, she said, and now her hair had matted into a disastrous 'bird's nest'.

When scientists examined the hair closely, however, they found that it showed all the signs of damage due to over-perming. Eventually the unfortunate lady admitted that she had tried to make her hair more interesting by perming it but she had had it done secretly and unprofessionally at home, so as not to flout the rules of her religion publicly.

Bird's nest hair always happens suddenly, and there is invariably a history of chemical

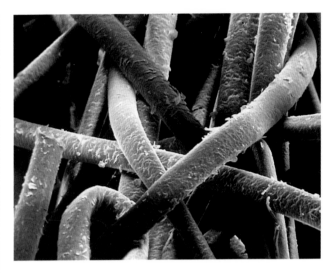

Severe matting, resulting in bird's nest hair

treatment. The treatment speeds up weathering and the hair rapidly starts to break down. As it does so the friction within it rises and the hairs begin to tangle together (though normally they don't form knots). This liability of wet hair to tangle is the reason why people with long hair should *never* pile it on top of their heads to shampoo it.

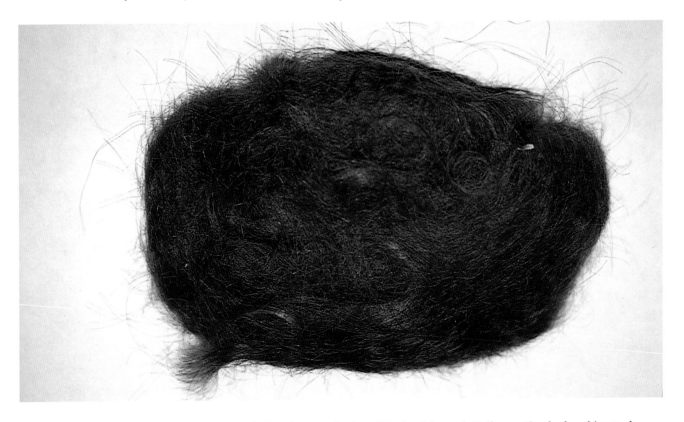

This hair became severely matted as a result of piling it up on the top of the head to wash it: the matting had nothing to do with any hair care product. The only possible course of action was to cut it off

5

Hair and scalp disorders

About this chapter ...

In this chapter we look at common disorders of the hair and scalp. Some of these, like dandruff and head lice, can be treated satisfactorily. For others, like the common baldness that affects up to 50% of men by the age of 50, there seems to be no effective treatment even though any number of remedies – both the seemingly logical and the completely illogical – have been proposed.

We need to understand the true causes of these problems. And it is just as important to know that some of the suggested treatments have no scientific basis at all.

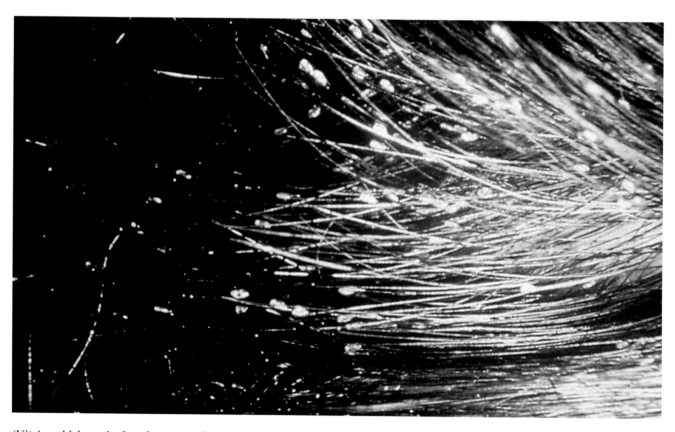

'Nits' – which are in fact the eggs or the young of the head louse – are one of the commonest of disorders of the hair, especially in children. The 'nits' seen here are the empty eggs, after the lice have hatched. Lice love long, clean hair, and do not like male hair after the teens

Hair loss

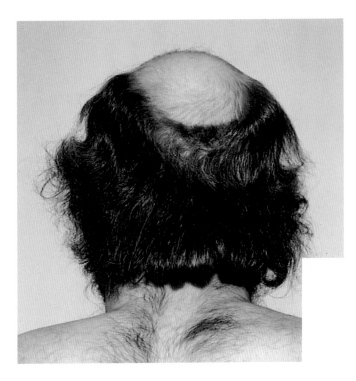

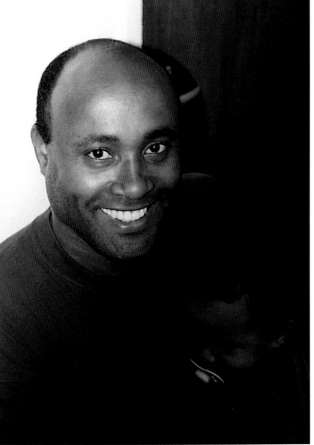

Hair loss is extremely common in both men and women; it is slightly more common in people with Caucasoid hair than in other types

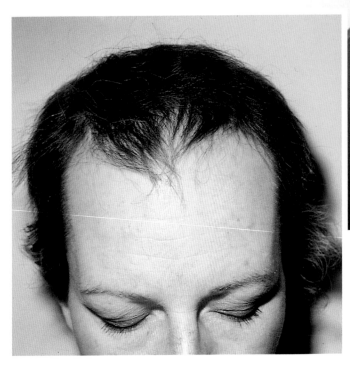

Hair loss

Natural shedding

As we saw in Chapter 1, all hairs naturally fall out at the end of the growing period. Everyone loses between 50 and 80 hairs a day. They tend to come out with brushing and shampooing. So if you wash your hair only once a week, it is perfectly in order for you to lose several hundred hairs at one go!

Sometimes, however, a person may start to lose more hairs than usual. If this hair loss is significant, and if it persists, then sooner or later the scalp may become visible through the thinning hair. The condition is called **alopecia**. The name comes from the Greek word *alopekia*, which means 'fox': foxes (and also dogs) sometimes suffer from bald patches due to an unpleasant disease called mange. (Fortunately, humans do not get mange!)

Baldness

The commonest kind of hair loss is simple baldness. Many people find this type of baldness embarrassing and distressing, but it is not a disease – it is a perfectly normal event. For thousands of years, however, it has caused concern and anxiety, and people have sought remedies and 'cures' without number, in spite of some of them being uncomfortable and even painful.

Baldness affects both men and women. It is much more obvious in men, however. By the age of 25, 25% of men have lost some of their hair, and the proportion rises to 50% by the age of 50. Many men accept, however reluctantly and vainly hoping that it may not be so, that they are likely to go partly or completely bald if their fathers have done so. They are right, in that baldness is genetically determined in both men and women. In women, however, baldness is not only unexpected, particularly in the twenties and thirties let alone later, but understandably unacceptable.

In men, baldness usually begins at the temples, above the forehead and at the crown of the head. In these areas the hair follicles of sufferers are genetically pre-programmed to revert from producing terminal hairs to producing vellus-like hairs. The growth phase of the hair (anagen) becomes shorter and shorter, with a greater proportion of hairs in the shedding (telogen) phase.

This change happens under the influence of male hormones (androgens) and can begin as early as the time of puberty or soon after, when androgen production in the body reaches a peak. Scientists call this kind of baldness **androgenetic alopecia** (meaning 'baldness due to androgens'). The eunuchs who served the harems of the east in days gone by never went bald!

Most women who come to dermatologists with hair thinning have androgenetic alopecia too. Baldness in women usually starts ten years or so later than in men, however. Fortunately for the sufferers, the amount of loss in women is differently distributed and less dramatic. The hairline usually remains intact and there is little or no loss at the temples. The illustrations show how hair loss develops over time in both men and women.

The patterns of baldness thus differ between men and women. Hair scientists speak of **male pattern baldness** and **female pattern baldness**. Occasionally, though rarely, women suffer from male pattern baldness and men from female pattern baldness.

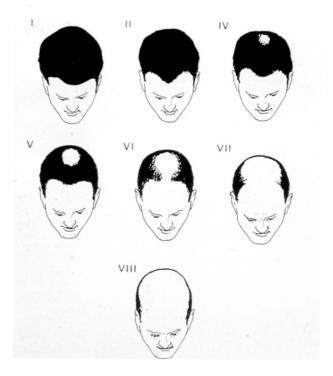

One pattern of hair loss, known as the Hamilton pattern, most usually seen in men

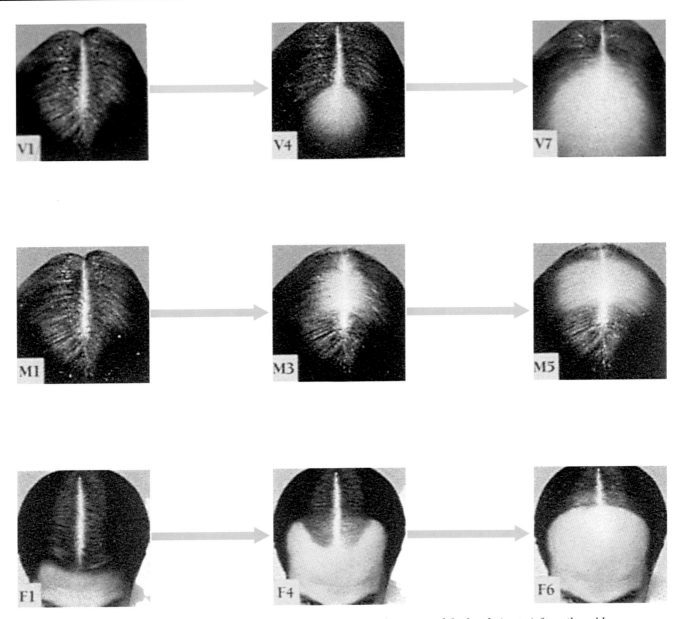

Progressive hair loss in Hamilton-type male pattern balding: (top) from the crown of the head, (centre) from the mid area, (bottom) from the forehead and temples

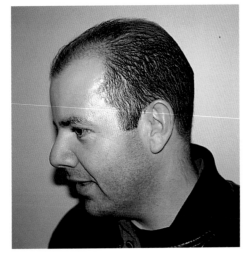

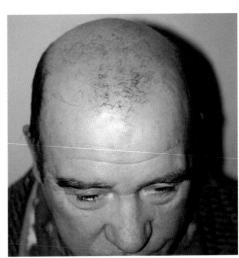

From this...   *...to this*

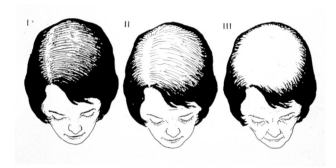

The Ludwig pattern of hair loss, which is most common in women

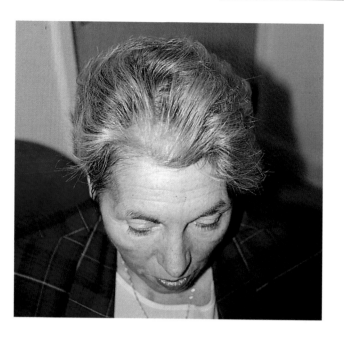

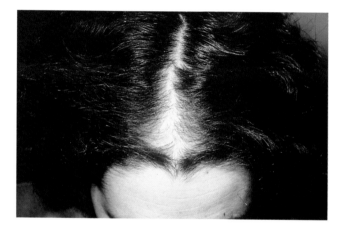

The typical Ludwig pattern of baldness, seen here in a young woman

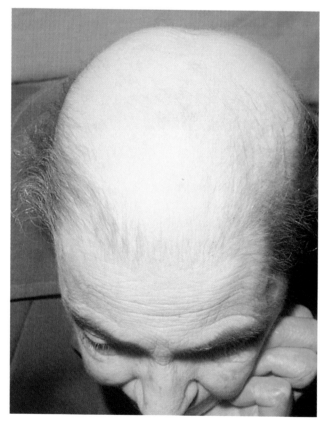

Female pattern balding: in spite of extensive hair loss, this lady has (just) retained her original hairline

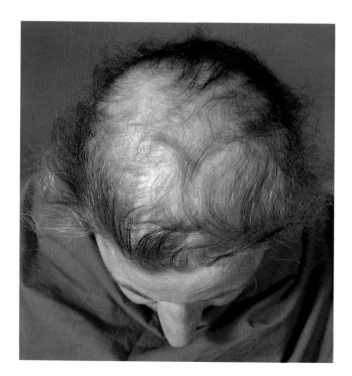

Extreme Ludwig pattern hair loss in an elderly lady

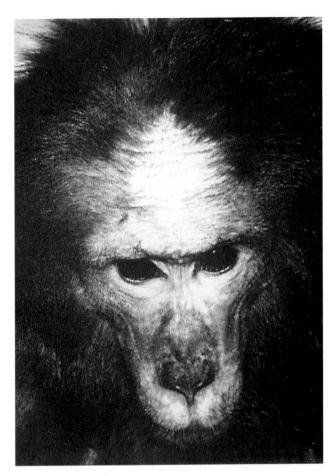

Apes suffer with alopecia too!

Humans are not the only primates in which baldness happens naturally at sexual maturity. Many orang-utans and chimpanzees of both sexes show some signs of baldness when they reach maturity.

Treatment for baldness

No one has yet achieved that longed-for prize so desperately sought, a certain cure for baldness.

A drug called **Minoxadil** is now available over the counter, or on private prescription, in the UK and in many other countries. The drug is applied to the scalp twice a day, but no guarantee of its effectiveness is offered. According to various experts it may at best stop the hair loss in about 80% of users; 30% will see some downy growth after three or four months or use, and a lucky 30% will see some visible re-growth of hair. It must be remembered that it has to be used continuously, for the rest of the user's life.

In the view of experts, most other so-called treatments are a waste of time and money. A great deal of research into the subject is going on, and other treatments may become available in the near future.

Diffuse hair loss

The second most common cause of hair loss is the general, or so-called **diffuse**, hair loss. In this condition the hair is shed from all parts of the scalp. A great deal of hair has to be lost before the effects become visible, however. The hair may fall during either the growing (anagen) or the resting (telogen) phase.

A sudden diffuse loss of hair may be both dramatic and distressing. One well-known cause of the loss of large amounts of hair is the drugs that are taken during cancer treatment, and in this case the hair is lost while it is in the growing phase. Fortunately the hair re-grows when the treatment is stopped.

Often women have some diffuse hair loss after the birth of a baby. During a pregnancy hair tends to grow well and to look healthy, under the influence of high levels of female hormones. It may in fact stay in the anagen phase throughout the pregnancy. When the baby is born this stimulation stops, and many of the follicles enter the catagen stage. Soon afterwards they enter the telogen phase in the normal course of events. They will be lost some two or three months later as the new hairs start to grow again. This is called **telogen effluvium**.

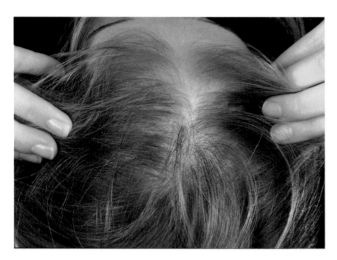

Two cases of telogen effluvium: the young woman above had a baby three months ago …

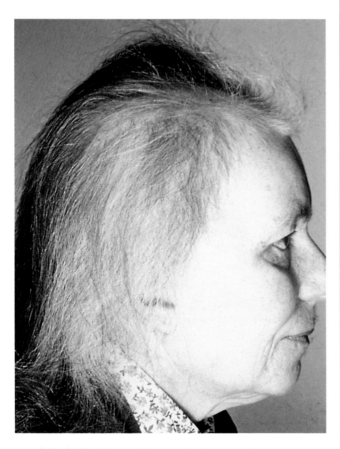

… while this lady's condition is due to iron deficiency

Other causes of diffuse hair loss include the following:

- high fever
- blood loss
- low levels of iron in the diet (possibly)
- starvation, or drastic dieting
- dental treatment or a surgical operation
- certain medicines
- disorders of the thyroid gland
- severe and prolonged emotional stress (possibly).

Anyone with diffuse hair loss, especially if it has begun fairly suddenly, should see a doctor who understands the condition, since the causes are not always easy to identify.

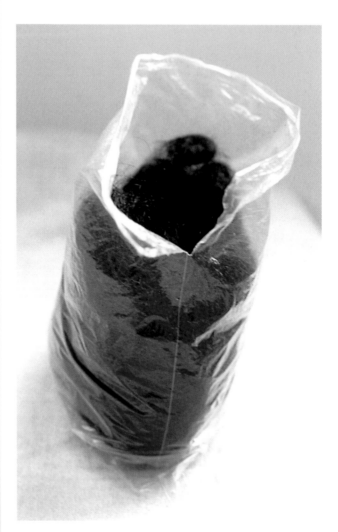

The amount of hair shed naturally by one person over one year

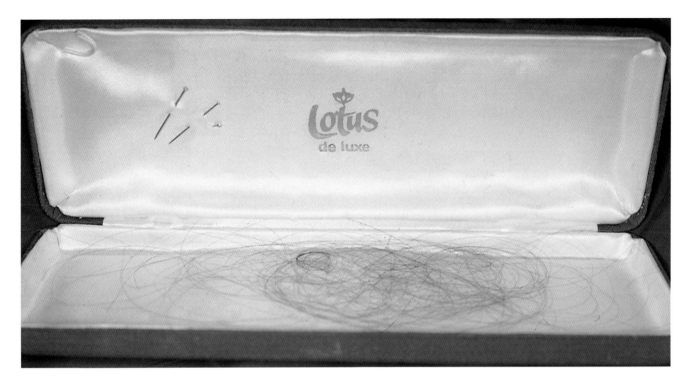

One day's natural hair loss

Bald patches

The sudden patchy loss of hairs may be due to a condition called **alopecia areata**. The condition can be recognised by examining the shed hairs under the microscope: in alopecia areata these look like exclamation marks. The sufferer may be only mildly affected, with thinning patches on the scalp, but occasionally the disorder becomes so widespread and severe that all the body hair is lost (see opposite page).

No one knows what causes alopecia areata. It usually disappears without treatment. Steroid injections given by a doctor may help in persistent cases of localised alopecia areata.

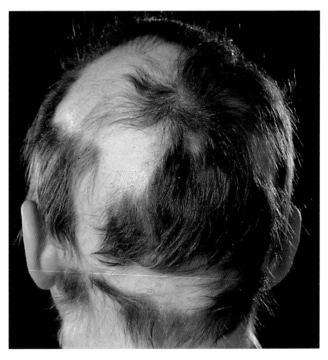

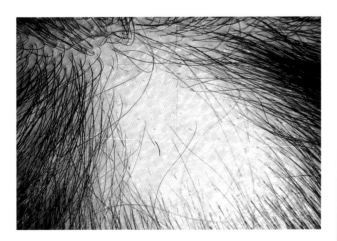

Classical alopecia areata, showing an isolated patch of almost complete hair loss

Acute and severe alopecia areata, in which hair over large areas may fall off at a touch

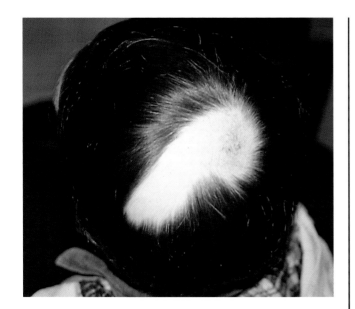

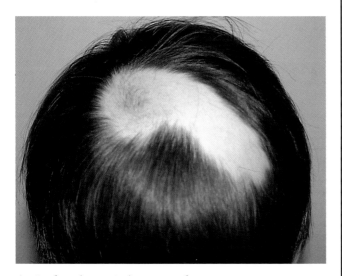

Acute alopecia areata in a young boy

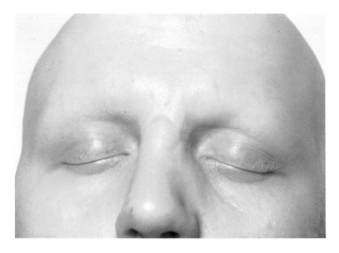

Alopecia totalis, a condition in which all the body's hairs are affected and the sufferer becomes completely hairless

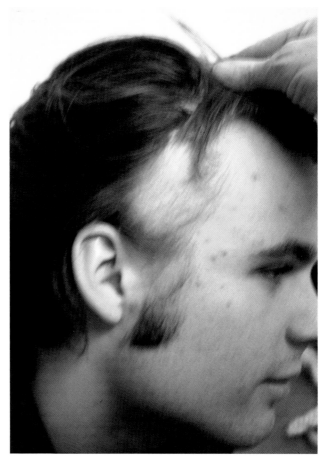

Acute alopecia areata in which – unusually – both temples are affected

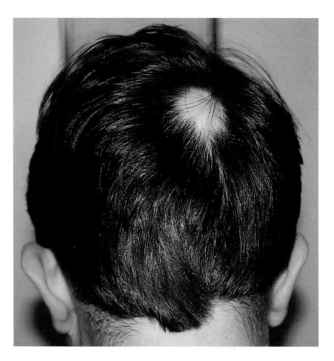

A typical case of alopecia areata seen in the salon

HAIR FACTS

Alopecia areata

Alopecia areata is not particularly rare: one person in every thousand can expect to suffer from it at some time in their lives.

Hair pulling

People with the condition called **trichotillomania** feel compelled to pull out their hair. The effects are seen on both the scalp and the upper eyelids. In the affected areas there are hairs of different lengths. When looked at under the microscope they show fractures.

The condition is common but not severe in children between the ages of two and six. In teenagers it is twice as common in girls as in boys, and can indicate the presence of a serious emotional difficulty.

Traction and trauma

So-called **traction alopecia** is seen in people whose hair is regularly subjected to strong traction (pulling). This can occur with ponytails or from backcombing or heavy-handed brushing. The braided styles and hair weaves often worn by Afro-Caribbean people put considerable tension on the hair, and can give rise to the condition.

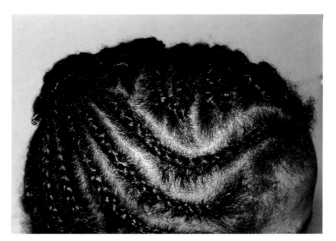

The effect of braiding, leading to traction hair loss

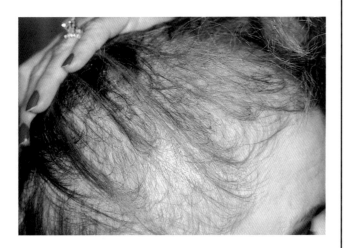

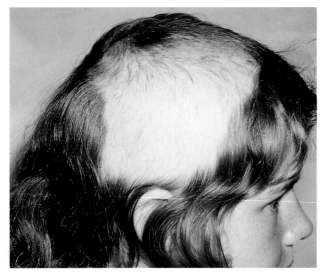

Typical cases of trichotillomania, due to repeated pulling out of hairs: the new hairs grow at different rates and therefore different lengths, as can be felt when the scalp is touched

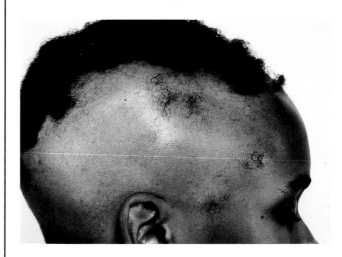

Hair loss due to traction and cosmetic abuse

Hair loss in children

We have already looked at several conditions which can lead to hair loss in children. Often an area of hair loss is seen at the age of two or three months, and this is quite normal. Sometimes the development of mosaic patterns of hair growth leads to apparent hair loss. Alopecia areata and trichotillomania are both seen from time to time in children.

In addition some children have a condition called **loose anagen syndrome**, in which the hair can be easily and painlessly pulled out. It is most common in fair-haired girls. It tends to improve as they grow older.

Hair shaft abnormalities

Sometimes hair is lost because the structure of the hair shaft is not normal. There are four main types of abnormality:

- fractures
- irregularities
- coiling and twisting
- extraneous matter.

Some of these characteristics are genetically determined (inherited). Others are the result of something that has happened during the person's life. Yet others are the result of an underlying disease. The photographs reproduced here show some examples. These cases are very rare, however: only about one person in every 10,000 is affected.

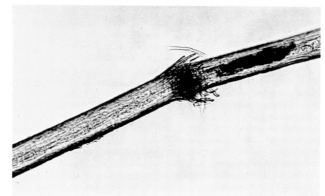

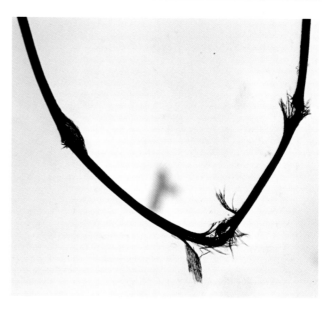

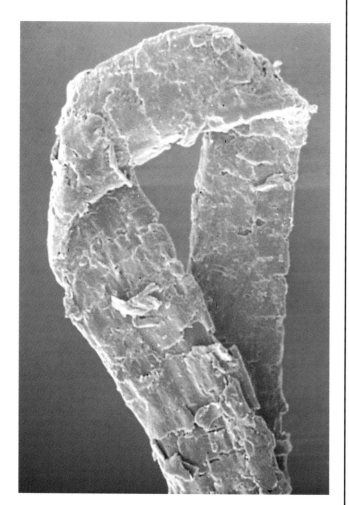

The condition known as trichothiodystrophy, which is a sulphur deficiency

The pictures above illustrate a type of hair malformation known as trichorrhexis invaginata

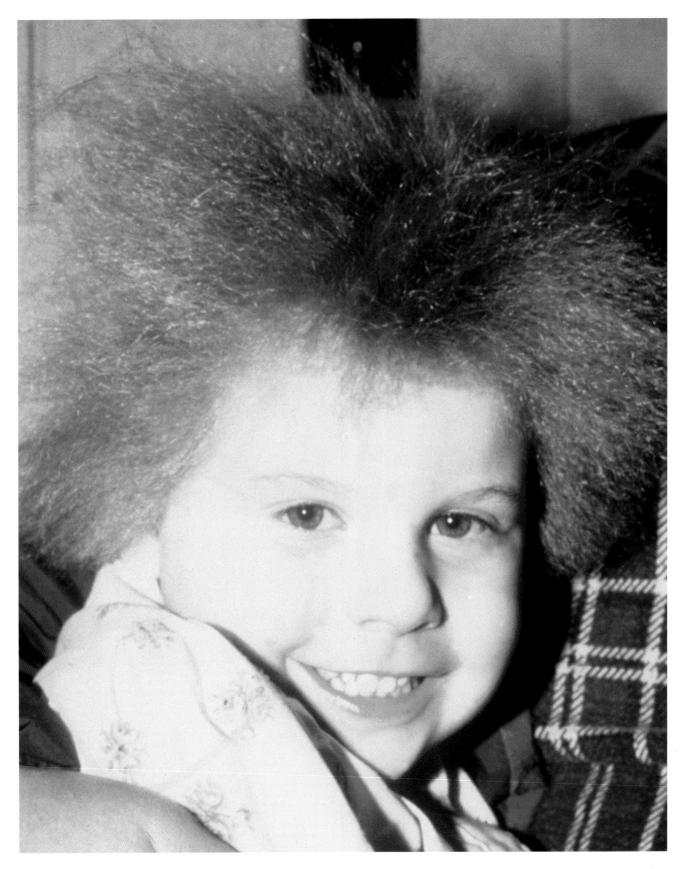

Cheveux incoiffables (literally, 'uncombable hair'): the hair shafts are congenitally abnormal (see opposite) and the hair stands straight up; it is vulnerable to damage and may break

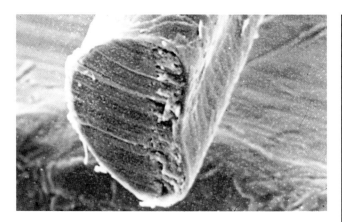

An abnormally shaped hair shaft associated with the condition known as cheveux incoiffables

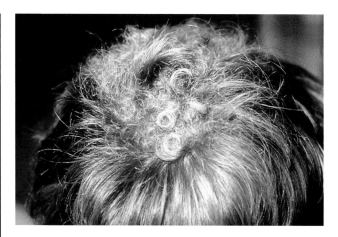

Woolly naevus is another congenital hair condition

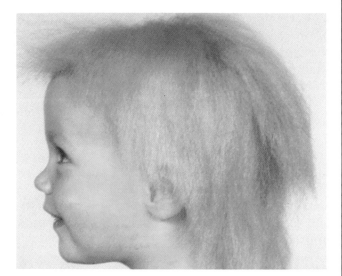

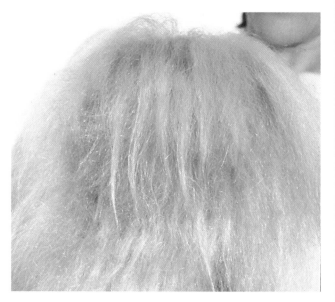

Two more examples of the congenital condition known as cheveux incoiffables

HAIR FACTS

Shampoos and hair loss

When people change their regular shampoo, mousse, conditioner or other hair product, they naturally give some extra attention to the condition of their hair and scalp. If they notice any improvement they give credit to the new product. Equally, if they notice anything amiss they blame the product. If they find that they are shedding hairs, they blame the product too – even if the loss has been going on for months. They can begin to believe they are going bald.

Research has shown that while many people understand that hair fall is a natural process in hair re-growth, others link it to the use of 'unsuitable' shampoos rather than to combing or brushing or to chemical changes like perming. Only a few people recognise factors like childbirth, medication, diet, genetic inheritance or illness as possible causes of hair loss, although all these are well known to hair scientists.

The fact is that shampoos do not cause hair to fall. Nor do they have any effect on the daily rate of loss, or on the rate of hair growth. Not surprisingly, more hair is shed on days when the hair is shampooed than on other days because of the simple mechanical action of washing the hair. Scientists studying different kinds of shampoos (including '2-in-1' products) could find no differences between their effects on hair loss.

Scalp disorders

The skin of the scalp is somewhat different from the skin elsewhere on the body. Not only does it have a very rich supply of grease from the sebaceous glands: it also carries follicles that produce long terminal hairs. Also both scalp and hair are more exposed to direct sunlight, cold and heat than most of the rest of the skin. And, of course, the scalp itself may be affected by many different cosmetic procedures, from simple shampooing to perming.

Hair stylists may see scalps that look scaly or inflamed. Problems concerning the skin of the scalp of course include some that affect skin elsewhere, and some that affect only the scalp area. Usually only the scalp is affected, but some of these conditions result in damage to the hair too, or even in hair loss.

Understanding these conditions and advising clients correctly is a vital part of client care.

Scaling conditions

Dandruff

The scientific name for dandruff is **pityriasis capitis**. The condition is all too familiar: about half of all Caucasians will have had dandruff to some degree before they are 20. In most of them it disappears after the age of 50 or so, however.

The top layer of the skin of the scalp (the epidermis), like that of skin everywhere else, consists of dead cells. These gradually wear away over time, and are replaced by cells from below. People with a greasy scalp seem more prone than others to this scaling away of the scalp.

Dandruff is associated with a tiny yeast called *Pityrosporum ovale*, which is normally present on the scalp all the time. In dandruff there is an increase in the regular loss of cells from the skin surface and they are lost more quickly: more cells are lost, and the yeast grows more rapidly. The cells may clump together to produce the all-too-familiar flakes of dandruff.

Simple treatments include the use of high-quality anti-dandruff shampoos, which contain substances that are active against the yeast. One of the best known is zinc pyrithione. These shampoos give all the cleaning and conditioning benefits that are associated with normal shampoos: they are not, as is often thought, harsh on the hair. Regular use of a shampoo of this type really helps to reduce the scaling.

Anyone with severe dandruff should be referred to a doctor.

Eczema and dermatitis

The most common problem of this kind is known as **seborrhoeic eczema**. It is accompanied by reddening of the skin, irritation and scaling. Sometimes it is associated with an unusually greasy scalp.

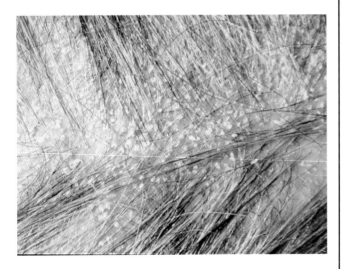

Dandruff can be an unpleasant and unsightly affliction

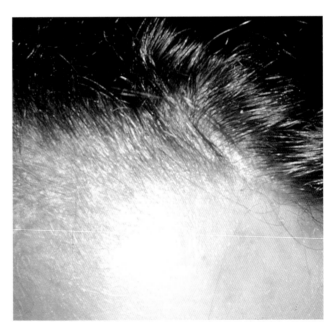

Seborrhoeic eczema

In babies, the condition known as **cradle cap** may be an early form of **atopic eczema**, which is a condition associated with hay fever and asthma.

Dermatitis of the scalp is also indicated by scaling and redness. If it is severe it may lead to hair loss.

Psoriasis

This distressing condition usually affects the skin of the inner knees and elbows, as well as that of the scalp. In some people the whole body can be affected. In a serious case the whole of the scalp may be covered by scales, and there may well be some hair loss.

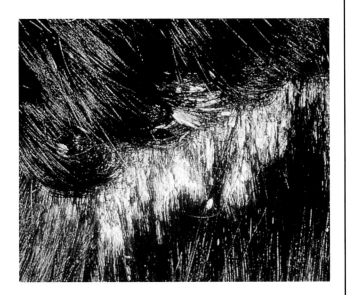

In psoriasis the hair takes on a coarse, asbestos-like appearance

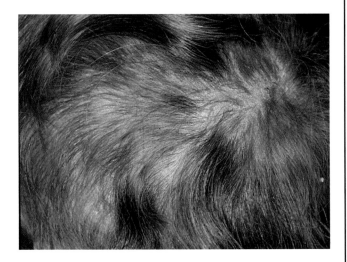

Hair loss in psoriasis

The condition can often be helped by coal tar pomades, but must always be referred to a doctor.

Infections

Impetigo

Impetigo is a bacterial infection of the skin, producing itching and weeping, crusted sores. It may affect the face as well as the scalp.

It is most often seen in young children, and may be associated with nits. It must be referred to a doctor for treatment.

Ringworm

Ringworm of the scalp is a fungal infection, which appears as pink, scaly patches on the skin. It is more likely to be caught from animals than from humans.

Any case of suspected ringworm should be referred to a doctor for medical treatment.

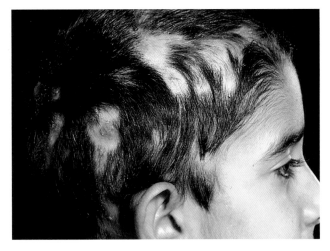

Ringworm of the scalp: sores and hair loss

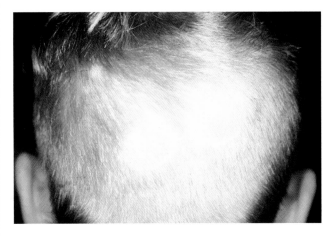

A severe attack of ringworm

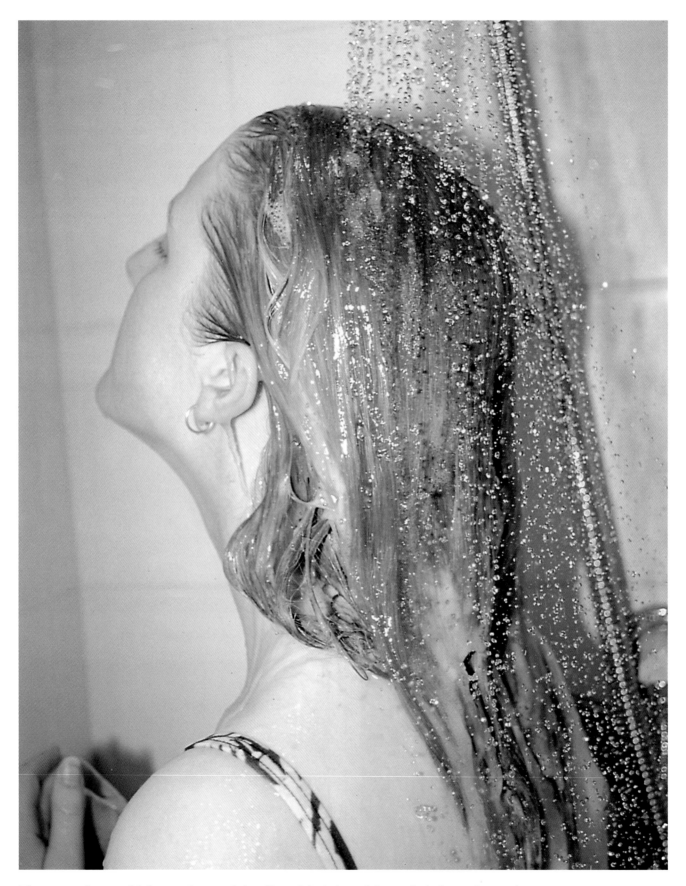

The secrets of successful shampooing: gentle handling of the hair, and thorough rinsing under running water

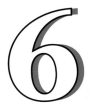

Hair care products

About this chapter ...

In this chapter we look at the major groups of hair care products that are sold for use at home and in the salon. We describe how these products are developed by the industry and how, before marketing, they are tested with the help of leading stylists and many of their clients.

We shall look at shampoos and conditioners, including '2-in-1' shampoo/conditioning preparations, and at the various styling products – setting lotions, mousses, gels and hair sprays.

Finally we explain the various steps in everyday hair care routines, and how to choose the right products to use on your own hair.

Shampoos

As a well-known hair scientist has said, *shampoos are simplicity out of complexity*. You could hardly guess what a complicated mixture is contained in that thick, fragrant liquid that you pour into your hand.

Shampoos have to be developed for different types of hair – normal, dry, greasy, permed, bleached and so on. Every shampoo has to be tested, not only as a formulation that is to be stored for months in a bottle or tube and then sold, but also as a product that is to be used on human hair and scalp.

In the laboratory, the experimental formulation is thoroughly tested on cut lengths of human hair before production is considered. The shampoo under test is applied to the hair and rinsed off, and an experienced technician judges the amount of tangling that results. This is only the start. Complex computer-assisted technology assesses many aspects of the product's performance.

If all goes well, the shampoo is evaluated in 'real life' conditions, on the hair of clients in salons. This is an essential part of testing, because it is the only way to judge whether the new product is acceptable to consumers. Only when these tests are completed safely and

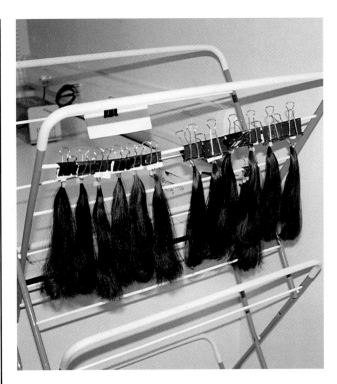

Test swatches of hair ready for evaluation

satisfactorily does the shampoo go on the open market for us all to try. This process may involve many thousands of tests and may take many months or years.

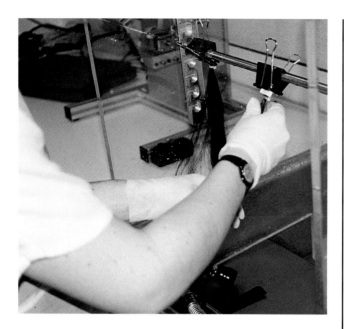

Product testing

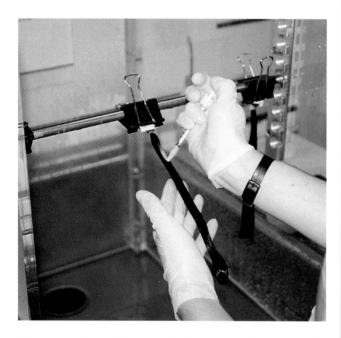

Testing new formulations in the laboratory with samples of human hair

The development of shampoos

The development of hair care products over the last few years has improved their quality enormously.

For many years, the main cleansing products – for hair as well as skin – were based on **soap**. But soaps have their disadvantages, especially in hard water. Soap will not lather well in hard water, and produces an unpleasant scum that cannot be rinsed away. If hair is washed with soap this scum deposits on the hair and leaves it looking dull and lifeless.

In modern shampoos soaps have been replaced by cleansers called **surfactants**. These lather well in all types of water and rinse off easily and completely. Most modern shampoos also contain some conditioning agents. The cleansing agents clean the hair and scalp, while conditioners make it easier to comb the hair while it is wet and give it volume without 'fly away' when it is dry.

Most people nowadays wash their hair more often than was usual even a few years ago. This has led to a great development of very mild cleansing systems. In addition, conditioners have been 'tailored' to suit different hair types, allowing users to match the level of conditioning to the requirements of the hair at that particular time.

There is no fundamental difference between the shampoos sold in salons and those sold in retail shops.

What is in a shampoo?

The ingredients in today's shampoos are all well known, thoroughly tested and officially approved. The skill and the science of the manufacturer is directed to developing products that best meet the needs of their users. Those needs extend to the care of *all* types of hair under *all* possible circumstances, including the hardness and temperature of water, and even abuse by the user!

A shampoo is a mixture of ingredients which can be classified according to the jobs that they do. In the European Union, all shampoos must carry a complete declaration of their ingredients on the packaging. The label doesn't always tell you why each ingredient is included, but you can often work it out for yourself.

Cleansing agents
The main reason why people use shampoos is to clean their hair. Grease (sebum) and dirt is removed from the hair and scalp by the surfactant system. The properties of the foam produced by the surfactants can be altered by the addition of what are known as 'lather boosters'.

HAIR FACTS

How often should I shampoo?

Hair *cannot* be washed too often!

Our ancestors washed their hair only rarely. We know that hair left unwashed for several weeks turns into a matted, smelly mess. We can only imagine the state of the scalps beneath those elaborate powdered wigs we see in portraits on the walls of stately homes!

This doesn't fit with our modern image of cleanliness and health. Hair can be washed every day, even several times a day if necessary. Today's shampoos do not damage hair. Their conditioning agents positively protect the cuticle against harm from brushing and combing.

So how often you wash your hair is a purely personal decision, one for you alone.

Conditioning agents
These condition the hair. Nearly all shampoos contain some conditioning agents. Some contain more than others do (see page 132).

Functional additives
These include ingredients that control the viscosity (thickness) of the shampoo. A shampoo that was too runny would be messy to apply, whereas one that was as thick as, say, toothpaste might be hard to spread over the hair.

Another kind of additive controls the pH of the shampoo. Usually shampoos are formulated to be slightly acidic, with a pH between 3.5 and 4.5.

Preservatives
A shampoo without preservatives would make a splendid breeding ground for germs of every kind. These could make the product 'go bad' or decompose, and they could present a considerable risk to health. Adding preservatives prevents problems like these.

Some of the preservatives you may see named on shampoo labels include sodium benzoate, parabens, DMDM hydantoin and tetrasodium EDTA. In spite of their rather alarming names, these are all safe, tested and approved ingredients.

HAIR FACTS

Surfactants

Surfactants are the essential cleaning substances in shampoos. Surfactant molecules have an unusual structure.

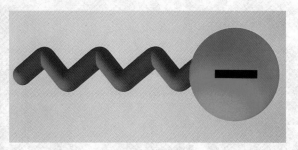

The structure of a surfactant molecule (diagrammatic)

One end of the surfactant molecule carries a tiny negative electrical charge. This end is soluble in water, and like water will not mix with oil or grease. The opposite end of the molecule is soluble in oily, greasy material and will not mix with water.

Surfactant molecules surround any fragments of greasy dirt they meet. The oil soluble parts of the molecules bury themselves in the grease. This leaves the water-soluble parts facing outwards from the fragment. As a result, the whole fragment becomes negatively charged.

This is useful because hairs themselves carry small negative charges on their surfaces. The two lots of negative charge tend to force each other apart – that is, the hair repels the dirt that was originally clinging to it!

Aesthetic additives
These are ingredients which are added to make the shampoo pleasant to use. They include colours, perfumes and pearlescing agents.

Medically active ingredients
Some shampoos contain active ingredients to treat medical conditions. For example, certain shampoos contain zinc pyrithione for the treatment of dandruff. Some contain panthenol, which is important for hair growth and which improves the moisture content of hair.

Just occasionally it can happen that shampoo is swallowed, perhaps accidentally, perhaps by an inquisitive child. For this reason every one of these ingredients is assessed, both alone and when combined with others, to check that it will not cause any harm in those circumstances.

HAIR FACTS

The principles of surfactants

All surfactants have the following features:

- They make the removal of dirt easier by reducing the surface tension between the water and the greasy matter on the hair.
- They produce foam (lather). The foam holds the bits of dirt in it, and stops them from being re-deposited on the hair.
- They stabilise the shampoo mixture, and hold the other ingredients in solution.
- They thicken the shampoo and make it easier to use.

Shampoos contain several surfactants – two, three or four. These give different types of cleaning, according to the type of hair. One commonly used surfactant, often mentioned on shampoo labels, is ammonium lauryl sulphate; another is ammonium laureth sulphate, which is milder.

The mildness of the surfactants is important for users who have sensitive skin and those who wash their hair frequently. By a 'mild' shampoo we mean one that does not damage the scalp, the hair or the eyes. But a user's assessment of 'mildness' can be different from those of the dermatologist and the hair scientist. Users sometimes assume that they can judge mildness by factors such as colour, perfume or whether or not the shampoo stings the eyes – even water can sting the eyes!

- For a shampoo to work efficiently, it must remove oils and grease from the hair.
- For a shampoo to be really mild, it must not remove the natural oils and grease from the skin.

Conditioners

As we have seen, most standard shampoos contain a certain amount of conditioning agents, so conditioning happens during shampooing anyway. Other preparations are applied after the shampooing is over. Which kind you choose is a matter of personal preference.

The molecules of most conditioning agents carry small positive electrical charges. As we have seen, hairs carry negative charges. The negative charges attract the positively charged molecules and these deposit on the hair, especially on areas where there is a degree of weathering. The immediate effect is that positive and negative charges cancel each other out, so reducing static electricity on the hair – and, of course, the 'fly away' that is associated with it.

The conditioners also help raised cuticle scales to lie flat against the hair surface. Not only does this improve the shine and lustre of the hair: the change in the hair surface enhances the depth and life of the hair colour too.

The smoothness of the conditioned hairs also means that detangling and combing the hair, both wet and dry, at once becomes easier. The hair becomes softer and more manageable. This is particularly important for dry, damaged or permed hair, to stop further deterioration.

'2-in-1' shampoos

'2-in-1' shampoos contain both cleansing agents and high levels of conditioning agents. These shampoos are everyday products now, but they created considerable debate when they were first introduced by Procter & Gamble in the 1980s. Scientists had believed that it was impossible to mix the cleansing and conditioning ingredients in a single bottle. However, it was made possible by adding special ingredients.

Nowadays all the major manufacturers produce '2-in-1' formulations, and over 20% of the shampoos sold are of this type. They basically rely on silicones, which are positively charged molecules derived from natural substances, to achieve conditioning in the way described above.

There is no question of conditioning agents building up on the hair if these shampoos are used repeatedly. Shampooing always removes the conditioning agents that were applied previously.

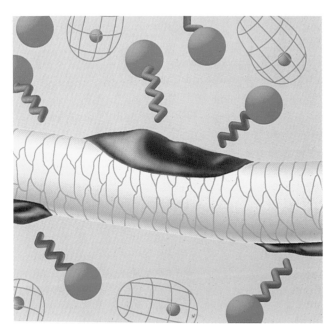

How 2-in-1 formulations work: (1) surfactant molecules (blue) and conditioner particles (pink) surround the hair; each conditioner particle is trapped inside a crystal 'cage'

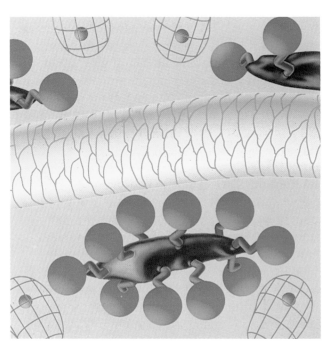

(2) The surfactant molecules are attracted to the dirt on the hair surface and lift it away, leaving the hair clean

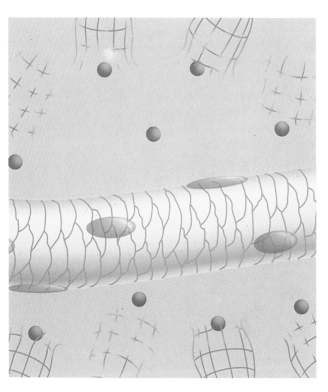

(3) When the hair is rinsed, the conditioner particles are released from their 'cages'; they are not washed away but, because of their electrical charge (+), they are drawn towards the (−) charges of the hair

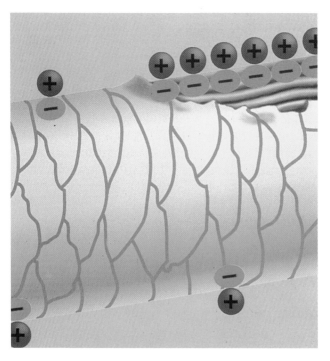

(4) They cling to the hair, smoothing out any roughness on the surface and protecting the cuticle

Styling products

These products are used to give the finishing touches to the chosen hair style, in order to get the final effect the user is looking for. Most are synthetic products, designed to make the hair thicker and firmer.

Setting lotions

These protect the hair from heat. Liquid lotions are designed to be used on wet hair. They give extra volume to the finished style.

Styling mousses

These can be used on either dry or wet hair, and are especially suitable for curly styles.

Gels

'Wet gels' give a glossy appearance to the hair. They work best with black hair.

Hair sprays

Hair sprays are generally used on dry hair, to hold and fix a style. A hair spray is a solution of a polymer (plastic) in a liquid.

The hair spray solution in the canister reaches the hair in the form of a fog of tiny droplets. When these strike the hair they join up, coating the hair thinly with the polymer. The spray dries very quickly, since the liquid evaporates almost at the instant it touches the hair. As it dries the polymer forms light welds or bonds between the strands of hair. It is these bonds that hold the newly created style in place.

Different types of hair spray are sold, for use on different types of hair. They differ in the formulation of the holding polymer used, and also in the way the spray is produced. Polymer sprayed on the hair in the form of large droplets gives more hold; it takes longer to dry, however, which leaves the hair feeling sticky for a while. It may also seem stiffer and rougher when it is dry. Smaller droplets give better feel, but a less firm hold. It is important to choose the right balance between hold and feel.

The more heavily the spray is applied, the stronger is the hold. But there is a definite trade-off: the build-up of polymer on the hair both looks and feels unpleasant. Some sprays feel sticky after even a fairly light application. A good spray will give both good 'hold' and good 'feel' without heavy or repeated application, and will be completely removed by shampooing.

Most hair sprays bond the hair strands into long, linear bundles – that is, they 'seam weld' the hair. But this structure is broken down as soon as a comb or fingers are run through it, or even in damp or windy conditions. A new innovation produces 'spot welds' rather than seam welds (see page 111). This reduces the volume of product on the hair. It also gives a softer hold and less damage to the cuticles when the hair is groomed.

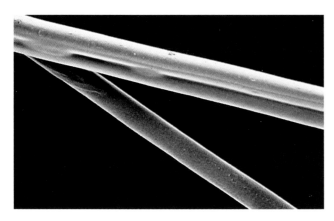

Traditional hair sprays produce seam welds between hairs, with rigid hold

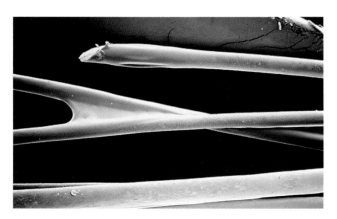

The latest 'Elastesse' technology: today's hair spray produces spot welds between the hairs, giving flexible hold and reduced product deposition

Hair care routines

Preventing damage

Hair is 'dead', and we cannot permanently repair any damage that happens to it. You only get one chance with your hair!

This is why it is so important to treat your hair properly, so as to *prevent* damage. One essential part of this is to adopt a good hair care routine, along the lines described below. Another is to keep chemical treatments like perming and bleaching to a minimum, as they can weaken the hair. Weak hair is easily damaged.

Choosing your hair care products

If you are to get the best possible results from your hair care routine, you need to choose the correct shampoo and conditioner for your hair type. How are you to decide which is your hair type?

Normal hair
Your hair is **normal** if:

■ it is neither greasy nor dry
■ it has not been permed or colour-treated
■ it holds its style well
■ it looks good and healthy most of the time.

If your hair matches any of these criteria, you should choose a shampoo and conditioner that are designed for normal hair.

Fine/greasy hair
Your hair is **fine** or **greasy** (or perhaps both) if:

■ it tends to be limp
■ it looks flat and lacks volume
■ it is difficult to manage because it does not hold a style
■ it soon gets greasy again after shampooing.

If you have hair of this kind, you will almost certainly have had problems with it. You will know all about the way in which greasy hair clings to itself and to your scalp, how the excess oil weighs the hair down and spoils your style, and how dust sticks to the grease so that your hair seems to be dirty only a day or two after it has been washed. You know that your hair's condition is due simply to your sebaceous glands being particularly active. But you can help it to improve.

Remember, sebum produced by your scalp does not spread itself over your hair by magic, or out of spite! It is spread by direct contact of the hair with your scalp. And something as simple as passing your fingers through your hair speeds up the transfer of the grease. So, after you have styled your hair, avoid fingering it or running your fingers through it. You can thus slow down the rate at which sebum collects on your hair, and it will not get greasy again quite so soon.

You should also wash your hair with a good cleansing shampoo specially designed for greasy hair, and use a special conditioner for greasy hair. This will improve the feel of hair that is greasy at the roots and dry at the tips, as well as protecting the hair from damage.

Dry hair
Your hair is **dry** if:

- it looks dull
- it feels dry or rough
- it tangles easily
- it is difficult to comb or brush
- it has been treated chemically (permed, bleached or coloured)
- it is liable to split ends
- it is dry and frizzy.

If your hair matches any of these criteria, you should choose a shampoo and conditioner that are designed for dry hair.

All these are just guidelines to help you choose the shampoo that is right for you.

Some people like to wash their hair every day or even more often, and choose a 'frequent use' shampoo. Most of today's shampoos are suitable for using as often as you could wish. This means that frequent users can choose products of the right type for their hair, and know that they can shampoo as often as they like.

People with hair and scalp problems like dandruff should choose shampoos that are specifically designed to treat their particular condition.

Regular hair care

Washing your hair
Everyone needs to wash their hair! But perhaps because everyone does it so regularly and so often, it is easy to forget how much damage you can do to your hair just in the simple shampooing and drying that has to be done over and over again. Here are some step-by-step guidelines for preventing unnecessary damage to your hair and keeping it healthy and shining.

1. Let your hair hang naturally while you wash it, either standing in the shower or with your head leaning over the bath.
2. Rinse your hair throughly with warm water to prepare it for shampooing.
3. Pour some shampoo into the palm of your hand. You will have to judge how much shampoo to use – you need enough to create a lather which will cover all of your hair.
4. Lather up the shampoo in your hand, and then apply it to your hair. Starting from the scalp, work the shampoo into your hair by gentle but thorough massage with your fingertips. Remember to keep your hair hanging naturally.

How not to …

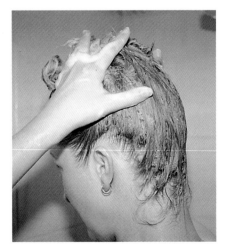

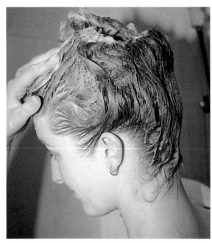

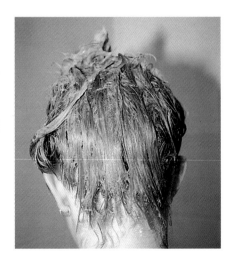

How not to wash your hair: piling it up on top of your head …

… and over-vigorous rubbing …

… leads to a mass of tangles!

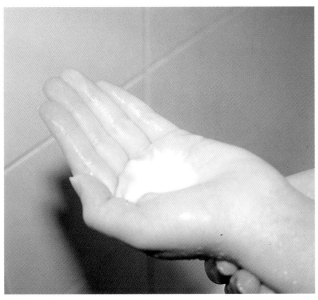

About the right amount of shampoo for long or medium-length hair

5. Rinse, letting the water run through your hair whilst you caress it downwards with your fingers. Be careful not to rub your wet hair too fiercely, as it is at this stage that hair is very easily damaged by friction.

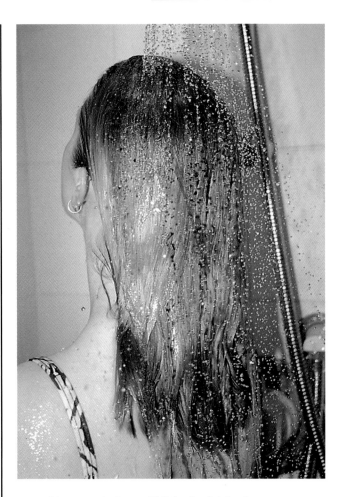

… and keep on rinsing until it is absolutely clean

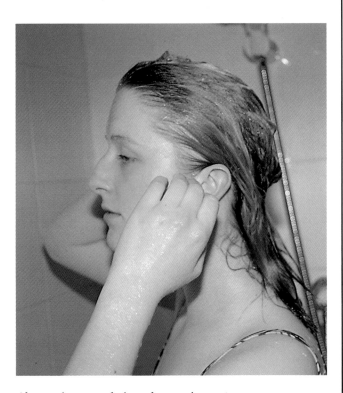

Always rinse your hair under running water …

Conditioning your hair

1. Make sure that you have rinsed all the shampoo from your hair.
2. Pour some conditioner into the palm of your hand.
3. Apply the conditioner to your hair and work it in gently but thoroughly with your fingertips – it must be spread evenly over your hair. Leave it to work for a minute or two.
4. Rinse off the conditioner, again allowing the water to run through your hair whilst you caress it gently downwards. Again, be careful not to rub your wet hair.

Drying your hair

1. Using a clean, dry towel, carefully pat your hair dry.

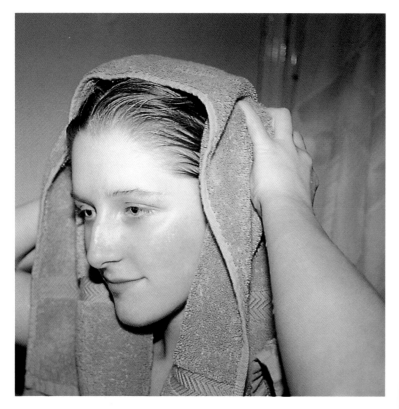

Drying hair correctly: again, don't pile it up, and don't rub it!

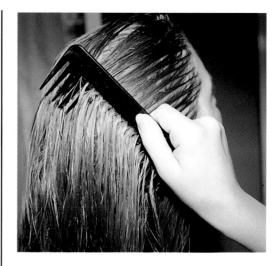

Gentle use of a wide-toothed comb prevents tangling and damage

2. While your hair is still damp, gently loosen out any tangles using a brush or a wide-toothed comb. Comb in downward strokes, starting near the tips and working your way upward towards the roots. This will help to keep the hair from splitting and breaking.

3. Apply a styling product such as a mousse or gel if you like, but don't use too much.

4. If possible, allow your hair to dry naturally.

Sometimes it may be impossible for you to find time to allow your hair to dry naturally, and you have to use a hair dryer. If so, here are some tips about using a dryer:

5. Only use the dryer on damp, towel-dried hair. Don't blow-dry hair when it is dripping wet!

6. Use the dryer cautiously, on the lowest speed and the lowest heat setting.

7. Keep the dryer moving constantly over your whole head. Don't concentrate the heat in one spot, as this can dry out the moisture from your hair and even damage it permanently.

8. Always switch off the dryer before your hair is completely dry.

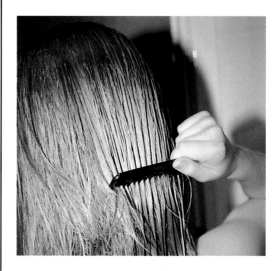

More gentle combing: correctly washed and conditioned hair does not tangle

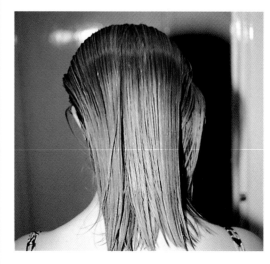

Almost done!

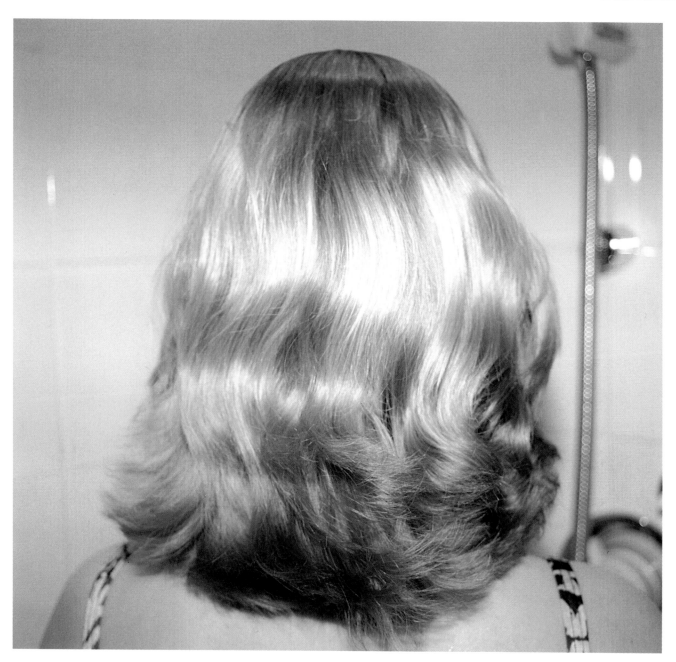

What we all aim for: smooth, healthy-looking hair that shines radiantly

We hope you have enjoyed reading this book and that it has proved useful in helping you to understand hair, hair science and hair care products.

To those of you who are or intend to be stylists and technicians, on behalf of Procter & Gamble Haircare Research Centre we wish you success in your chosen career. And to all of you, we wish good luck with your hair!

Index